PENGUIN BOOKS

MASTER THE MARATHON

Ali Nolan is a journalist and writer based in Utah. As the former features editor and a current contributor for *Runner's World*, she is active in empowering women in the running world, having spoken at the Under Armor Women's Panel, Donna Marathon Pre-race Dinner, and other events. She has completed two road marathons, a trail marathon, and other races.

MASTER
THE
MARATHON

The Ultimate Training

Guide for Women

ALI NOLAN

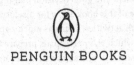

PENGUIN BOOKS

PENGUIN BOOKS

An imprint of Penguin Random House LLC
penguinrandomhouse.com

All photographs courtesy of the author.

LIBRARY OF CONGRESS CATALOGING-IN-PUBLICATION DATA

Names: Nolan, Ali, author.
Title: Master the marathon : the ultimate training guide for women / Ali Nolan.
Description: New York City : Penguin Books, 2021.
Identifiers: LCCN 2021012072 (print) | LCCN 2021012073 (ebook) |
ISBN 9780143135487 (paperback) | ISBN 9780525507130 (ebook)
Subjects: LCSH: Women long-distance runners—
Training of. | Marathon running—Training.
Classification: LCC GV1065.17.T73 N65 2021 (print) |
LCC GV1065.17.T73 (ebook) | DDC 796.42082—dc23
LC record available at https://lccn.loc.gov/2021012072
LC ebook record available at https://lccn.loc.gov/2021012073

Printed in the United States of America

Set in Minion Pro
Designed by Cassandra Garruzzo

Outdoor recreational activities are by their very nature potentially hazardous. All participants in such activities must assume the responsibility for their own actions and safety. If you have any health problems or medical conditions, consult with your physician before undertaking any outdoor activities. The information contained in this guide book cannot replace sound judgment and good decision making, which can help reduce risk exposure, nor does the scope of this book allow for disclosure of all the potential hazards and risks involved in such activities. Learn as much as possible about the outdoor recreational activities in which you participate, prepare for the unexpected, and be cautious. The reward will be a safer and more enjoyable experience.

*This book is dedicated
to my grandmother, Maria Campo*

CONTENTS

FOREWORD

When you tell someone you are a runner, two questions immediately follow: "What is your mile time?" and "Have you run the marathon?" The mile and the marathon are the events in distance running that matter the most; they are running's "sexy" events.

The mile is the perfect short story: every detail matters and there's not a second to waste. You come off the start line at a hot pace and keep that rhythm high as lactic acid builds in your muscles and sears your lungs. It's four perfect laps of suffering that are over in an instant. As a young runner, the mile captured my heart. The speed, the burn, the pain that happened over the distance made me feel alive.

I spent much of my early running career hanging on to the idea that I was made for speed. I looked at longer distances as a cop-out of "real" racing. Longer distances were the polar opposite of feeling alive: they were hours of slow running where you battled off a long, slow death. Not for me, I had decided.

The marathon is a completely different beast from the short story that happens on the track. It's an epic tale that unfolds over thousands of pages. It should come as no surprise that the origin story of the marathon comes from a Greek legend; the event is rooted in allure and history. Legend has it that Pheidippides ran the roughly twenty-five-mile route from Marathon to Athens to announce the Greek victory over the invading Persian army. Upon reaching the Athenian agora, Pheidippides announced, "Rejoice! We conquer," then promptly died from exhaustion. Naturally, this has become something that we mortals feel we must replicate and put to the test. Can we perform such an amazing feat? Can we master the marathon?

After departing college and spending those years as a track runner, trying to master the art of speed, I finally gave in to the challenge of the marathon. Feeling alive on the track had been fun, but who wouldn't want to write their own epic tale of how they fended off death by exhaustion? The idea of pouring all my energy into 26.2 miles of road stretched out in front of me seemed simultaneously daunting and thrilling. There's so much distance to cover. So much to learn. So much time for everything to go wrong, or just right. This was a chance to learn an entirely new sport.

I signed up for my first marathon in the spring of 2007, and I buried myself in the training. I strung together weeks, and then months, of the highest mileage of my life. I conquered twenty-mile-long runs for the first time. I learned about cumulative fatigue. I prepared my mind. I trained my gut because in the marathon, that's a thing that needs to be trained, too—who knew?

I lined up for the 2007 Boston Marathon in nor'easter conditions, feeling like I had prepared for everything that the event could possibly throw my way. Boy, was I wrong. I battled through the conditions and competed with some of the best runners in the country and the world and finished a respectable eighteenth place. I loved every second of the race, and as it was unfolding, I knew that as prepared as I thought I was, I had only scratched the surface of understanding the event. I crossed the finish line and I was hooked. It took me only one run over the fabled 26.2-mile distance to realize: track running can make you feel alive, but the marathon can transform your life.

The puzzle of the marathon has kept me coming back to it for years. In the process of trying to put together my perfect race, I've managed to run myself onto two U.S. Olympic marathon teams, finish in the top five at nine Abbott World Marathon Majors races, and even win the Boston Marathon in some of the worst racing conditions in the history of the sport. You might think I have the whole distance figured out, but I don't. In fact, every time I complete a training block and finish a race, I'm taken aback by all the new things I've learned and what I still haven't gotten just right.

The deeper I get into the marathon training game, the more I realize that nailing the details can make or break your experience. The marathon is chess, not checkers. If we're fine-tuning details, shouldn't we have a resource that is tailor-made for women's specific needs? After all, as environmental exercise physiologist and nutrition scientist Dr. Stacy Sims says, "Women are not small men." Having *Master the Marathon* as a resource designed specifically for women is going to help us find our proper paces, necessary fueling needs, optimal mind-set, and more by using the details in our life and physiology that make us unique. Most important, this guide is going to provide you with the practical tools to help you become a better version of yourself. In the following pages you'll encounter tips from the foremost female experts and coaches in running. Use their wisdom and motivation as you work through your own marathon journey and craft your own epic version of the marathon tale.

DESIREE LINDEN

MASTER
THE
MARATHON

CHAPTER 1

A GUIDE, JUST FOR YOU

So you want to run a marathon? What are you thinking? Do you really want to pour every last ounce of energy you have in your reserve into a monthslong process that culminates in your sweating, crying, and belching your way across a marathon finish line? The answer is, of course, yes. If you've been there before and you're hooked, know that I understand. If this is your first, you've entered a whole new dimension of self-imposed human suffering. And you know what? It's amazing.

During this process, you'll get input from a variety of people. Your friends, your colleagues, your great aunt Norma—people who have hardly walked outside to take their trash out, let alone run a marathon—will want to offer unsolicited advice. They all mean well. They'll probably also tell you that running the marathon in and of itself is an accomplishment.

Sure, I think we can all agree that running 26.2 miles is a huge athletic achievement. But, my dear marathoners, I have a question for you. If you're going to dedicate months of training to a single day in your life, don't you want to put everything you've got into making it the best dang race ever? Shouldn't your goal be to finish knowing that you did everything in your power to kick the marathon's butt? Yeah, I thought so. It's time to live up to your truest potential. Guess what? You're ready.

Training for 26.2 is something almost otherworldly. The process is immersive, focused, and can at times lift you out of your humanoid self and onto a plane of the divine. At other times, you might feel stomped on, used up, and so freaking tired. And yet you relish the agony because, despite the physical pain, excitement builds within you. At the end of all the work, you will line up and run 26.2 miles. It will be hard, but it will also be spectacular.

WHY DO WE NEED A MARATHON TRAINING GUIDE SPECIFICALLY FOR WOMEN?

As of 2020, only 0.5 percent of people in the U.S. could say that they have completed a full marathon. Women represent 45.7 percent of runners within that tiny group. This number—which shows women making up nearly half of the marathoning population—amazes me. Female athletes have come so far in such a short span of time. As recently as 1966, women were forbidden to run 26.2-mile races. Professionals believed it was physically impossible and dangerous for women to run anything more than a mile and a half. (One common myth was that if women ran any farther, our uteruses would just fall out.) But as with many other barriers women have faced over the course of history, we fought our way in.

In 1966, Bobbi Gibb snuck onto the Boston Marathon course and became the first woman to run the full course. When Gibb talks about running, it's clear that the sport always meant more to her than racing or competing. She ran for the beauty of it—to be at one with nature and herself. There was no ego involved, no obsession about her times. Her idea of a good run was looking into the distance at a mountaintop and spending the whole day running to the summit. The Boston Marathon was the only marathon she knew about. She lived in Massachusetts, and in 1964 she happened to see a portion of the race while she was on her own run. When she decided to start training for it, she didn't know that it was only for men. Her desire to run it, at the time, was not about making a statement or starting a movement. She admits she was naive—in both running and the politics of sport. She ran in nurse's shoes. She did not have a training manual. Her boyfriend at the time would take her out on his motorcycle and then drop her off in the middle of nowhere, and she would joyfully run home.

By 1965, she was strong enough to run forty miles at a time. In 1966, she wrote to the Boston Athletic Association to apply to run the marathon. Will

Cloney, the race director, rejected her application. He wrote back to her and said that women were not physiologically capable of running 26.2 miles and that the rules said they were not allowed to run.

She was shocked. Of course it was possible for women to run 26.2 miles. Bobbi continued to train, now aware that this was bigger than her and her ambition to run the marathon.

The day of the race, her mom dropped her off at the start. She hid in the bushes until the gun went off, then jumped into the pack. Her final time was three hours and twenty-one minutes. On the Boston course, which is notoriously hilly and difficult, this is an incredible feat, and she finished ahead of two thirds of the field. Bobbi set the sport free that day, though there would be struggles for equality in the sport for years to come.

In fact, the next year, women were still not allowed to run the Boston Marathon. Bobbi ran without a bib again. But another woman, Kathrine Switzer, applied to run the marathon under a pseudonym, a man's name, to conceal her identity. She was assigned the bib number 261 and arrived at the start proudly sporting it across her chest. Bobbi's under-the-radar run had gained press attention and even support from some runners, and the marathon officials turned a blind eye. But it seemed that Kathrine's open defiance of the rules posed a real issue for the race director, Jock Semple. He charged out onto the racecourse and tried to rip the bib from Kathrine's sweatshirt.

"A big man, a huge man, with bared teeth was set to pounce, and before I could react he grabbed my shoulder and flung me back, screaming, 'Get the hell out of my race and give me those numbers,'" Switzer writes in her memoir, *Marathon Woman*. "Then he swiped down my front, trying to rip off my bib number, just as I leaped backward from him."

Another runner, a man Switzer knew, punched Semple to get him off her. The altercation was caught on camera by journalists, who were fascinated that a woman would even attempt to run the distance. Bobbi Gibb's and Kathrine Switzer's boldness helped pave the way for female runners, but it took time.

Nowadays, female distance runners are finally getting the positive attention and respect they deserve. The elite and sub-elite women are getting faster and faster. Many of them (who are experts you'll find in these chapters) have focused on what makes female runners different and used that information to enhance their abilities.

I want to reiterate my previous sentence: female runners are different from male runners. For too many years, women runners have followed the men's playbook. Most of the popular and respected training manuals are by men. And indeed, they are experts when it comes to how men can and should train. But due to some of the biological differences between women and men, there are also differences in the way that women and men run.

We have smaller hearts, which means our intake of oxygen is less than men's, which contributes to our (on-average) slower speeds. While this is just a biological difference—not an inherent flaw—women can take action to boost their aerobic capacity, and you will find a great deal of training to do so in this book.

In terms of strength, a study in the *Journal of Applied Physiology* found that men had an average of twenty-six pounds more skeletal muscle mass than women. Women also exhibited about 40 percent less upper-body strength and 33 percent less lower-body strength, on average. Women can benefit and see faster results when they integrate a targeted strength program into their marathon training plan.

The majority of recreational runners are heel strikers, which means our heels are the first thing to touch the ground. Forefoot striking (landing more in the center of your foot) is optimal. More women are heel strikers than men, and while that doesn't bode well for momentum, it isn't the worst thing in the world. But we do have to take extra care of our feet, ankles, and lower leg muscles.

None of these things makes us worse or better runners—we are different. Well, wait. We are better at endurance and pacing, according to a study out of Marquette University.

All this is to say: Women shouldn't follow the exact same training regimen as men. We need training programs tailored to our bodies—to our unique strengths and weaknesses—so that we can avoid injuries and run at our peak. The programming in this guide is made especially for women.

HOW TO USE THIS BOOK

My hope is that this little book will guide you through the entire marathon process. I want to help you through the good and the bad, the hard and the exhilarating, and then slowly but surely become your BFF. OK, but really, I just want to inspire your running. I hope that you will feel motivated and strong from the day you decide to run a marathon to the finish line.

With that being said, I want to talk to you about the process as a whole. Some of you who are reading these words have never run a mile in your life. For others, your next marathon will be your tenth or fiftieth. My advice to all of you is the same. If you are looking to unlock the secret to running your best race, give yourself time. This is a process that will affect your whole life and will result in positive change, if you let it.

Never fool yourself into thinking that you're only in this for the time leading up to the race. You're a runner. Your journey is everlasting. Mastering the marathon is a lifelong pursuit that you can and will achieve over and over again at different levels. It's a beautiful process with ups and downs, hard weeks and off weeks. You chose this running life. Every mile you put into it will give you something in return.

If you haven't already, it's time to start thinking about your training holistically. There are five elements that go into a successful marathon: running, mentality, strength training, nutrition, and recovery.

Many athletes have the running part down. But throughout my time researching, reporting on, and participating in marathons, I have found that most women, myself included, are not paying attention to all the other essential components. We should place equal value on these parts because they all play a role in race-day performance. The obvious place to start, believe it or not, isn't running. It's your mind.

FIRST STEP

When you've decided to run a marathon, perhaps the most important thing you must do—before stepping out onto the road or jumping on a treadmill—is to ask yourself: Why? Why do I need to devote my time, body, energy, and mind to an endeavor that is so grueling that only 1 percent of the entire human population has put themselves through it?

I want to be real with you. If you're a first-time marathoner, then you have to know that this gets really hard. The training is difficult. It will consume parts of your life. At times, no matter how fit or focused you are, you will be tired, sore, achy, and ravenously hungry—and you will still have to live your normal life.

If you are an intermediate or advanced runner who is leveling up her time goal, you might know just how devastating it is when something derails a training cycle. If you've never suffered through pool jogging while waiting for a shin splint to heal, then you probably can't understand the agony and anxiety that being pulled away from a traditional running plan causes.

What I'm trying to say is that stuff happens. Life happens, pain happens, and unless you have a really solid reason to run this marathon, the marathon might steamroll over you.

When we talk about goals, we sometimes just think in terms of time or outcome. Newbies usually say, "I just want to cross the finish line." Experienced marathoners might say, "I want to run under four hours" or "I want to qualify for Boston." These are extrinsic goals, which are awesome! I love them—everyone loves them! But they don't necessarily work 100 percent of the time.

Let's say, for example, you make it all the way to the start line and you've followed all the instructions in this guide, but a thunderstorm rolls through just as you hit mile eighteen, and the marathon organizers have to herd all the remaining racers off the course and you can't finish. Does that mean that you failed? Is crossing an arbitrary line the only measure of success?

And for all of you who want to BQ,* you know how tough this is. You know that even on the best day, with the perfect training cycle, there are myriad obstacles that could prevent you from achieving your goal. For example, what if an unscheduled train rolled through a railway crossing and just stopped . . . for several minutes . . . in the middle of the racecourse?

---

* BQ stands for "Boston qualifying" time—it is shorthand for running a marathon time that would qualify you for the Boston Marathon. The times are ridiculously challenging and vary by age range. The Boston Athletic Association updates the qualifying times every few years to reflect the ever-improving times of marathoners.

We all need extrinsic goals. They help us achieve our dreams and give us much-needed ego boosts. But setting and focusing on intrinsic goals will guide us through our training. Ideally, your intrinsic goals will be what leads to the extrinsic accomplishment.

Here are the differences:

Extrinsic Motivation	Intrinsic Motivation
Winning	Fun
Time goals	Growth
Prizes or awards	Passion
Social praise and attention	Self-worth

If you are running for extrinsic goals exclusively, it's hard to persist and improve. If running is just the instrument that leads to fulfillment, and not enjoyment in itself, then I must tell you, it will take an exhausting amount of focus and determination to make it through an entire training period. And at the end, even if you achieve that goal, you might feel deflated or empty.

Some people who aspire to run a marathon will stick to their guns and do the training because they want to challenge themselves. Others will give up on day two because they don't have meaningful motivation. Often what people in the latter camp are really seeking is social praise and attention, and when they realize that running kind of sucks, especially for beginners, and that they can't just pick up a twelve-week marathon-training PDF and expect to be race ready in three months, they quit.

Anyway, I bet if you're reading this book, you already have the meaningful motivation it takes to train and run a marathon. But you might have some tricky extrinsic goals that could actually stand in your way instead of propelling you forward. There are a few common ones for people who sign on to run a marathon:

Weight loss
Charity
New Year's resolution
Personal record (PR)

These aren't the worst goals! But we can do better. Let's examine each of these goals more thoroughly.

Weight Loss

We'll get more into weight loss in our chapter on nutrition, so for now, let's just say that the number on the scale is not a metric we can trust. This is an easy one to update, though:

I'm running a marathon for weight loss. → **I'm running a marathon** to become a physically and mentally healthier version of me.

Charity

Charity is a noble reason for running and a pretty decent why. Charity is one of those that I could count as either an extrinsic or an intrinsic motivation, depending on how you look at it. I mean, it is absolutely beautiful to dedicate a race to a worthy cause and to be able to draw on that reason while you're grinding. But girl, that's still your body out there on the line. Make it personal to ensure you're benefiting from the experience too! Yes, you're allowed to have multiple intrinsic goals.

I'm running a marathon for charity. → I'm dedicating a race to the ASPCA in honor of my rescue dog Ollie. In the process, I hope to fall in love with running, mostly so I can go back to the shelter and run all the adoptable dogs around, and then maybe bring them home.

Wait, let me try that again:

I'm running a marathon for charity and for self-discovery and passion.

New Year's Resolution

Do I even need to tell you about the day in February where New Year's resolutions go to die? If you're thinking you are going to start a training cycle right after the holidays, when most of the United States is covered in ice and when your local gym is crammed with people, then you better hope you can identify a couple more intrinsic motivators, because otherwise that dream will be long gone.

I'm running a marathon because it's my New Year's resolution. → **I'm running a marathon** to find inner strength! I want to get healthier and stronger!

Personal Record (PR)

Running a personal record (PR), sometimes called a personal best (PB), means that you have bested every race time you have run before. Now, this one is really tricky for me, and I think that running a PR could potentially be considered either an extrinsic or an intrinsic goal, because it's about becoming a better version of yourself and growing. But to set this as an intrinsic goal, you need to know yourself well. Can you look beyond the end result to find joy in the process? Then fine, you're basically self-actualized. Your less-evolved sisters struggling with perfectionism are just over here envying you. If you're a tad less progressed, then let's shift that PR goal.

I'm running a marathon to set a PR. → **I'm running a marathon** to improve my running, strengthen my running weaknesses, finish a race feeling fresh and energized.

It's not that hard to find internal motivations, but it's crucial to do so before you even think about registering for a race. That's because when your alarm rings to rouse you from your slumber at five forty-five on a cold autumn morning and you know you're facing an eighteen-miler, and it's late into your training cycle right in the not-so-sweet spot where you're hitting about forty-five total weekly miles, so your body feels like it's basically just a human-shaped pile of oatmeal mush, and you finally wake up but now you're struggling to put on your sports bra because your underarms are chafed, and you can't find your left running shoe, and so you sit down at the foot of your bed and think about quitting, that's when you think of your "why." And you realize, there is no quit in you.

Hopefully with this guide, no morning will ever suck that badly. But just in case, find your why. Then write it on a piece of paper and tape it to the mirror where you brush your teeth in the morning.

At the beginning of a new training cycle, when I'm at the point where I need to find my why for a particular race, I write out all the reasons I run. I run because it gives me an incredible feeling of freedom. I run to learn something new about myself and how much I can handle every race season. I run because I love spending time with my running friends. The list goes on. Your list will likely give you insights into the real reasons you have for running a marathon. Write them out here:

I run because . . .

1. _____

2. _____

3. _____

4. _____

5. _____

Intrinsic goal setting is particularly important for intermediate and advanced runners. So many of us get lost in the data of our paces, splits, and PRs. Setting a PR is exhilarating, but it must be secondary to our true motivation for running. Those numbers don't determine our self-worth. Only when we set aside the external will our egos be quiet and calm enough to let our bodies perform at their respective peaks.

CHAPTER 2

PLANNING YOUR TRAINING CYCLE

N ow let's talk about physical training. You probably want to know how long you should give yourself before your first (or next) race. Like many things, it will depend on your running history. An intermediate or advanced runner should plan for a race that is at least six months away. A casual runner should plan for a race that is about a year away. And someone who is completely new to running should plan for a race that is about sixteen months away.

Sixteen months—man, I know that sounds like a long time. Here's the deal. When you give yourself time to learn about your body's reaction to running, you are more apt to make training a whole-body experience. If you have your nutrition, strength, mental game, and recovery process keyed in, you will go into the actual training strong and prepared. You'll need to make a few adjustments, but you'll likely face less pain and turmoil than someone who just woke up and decided to run a marathon.

My first marathon, the Marine Corps Marathon, was a big goal—a goal that I wanted to achieve for approximately five minutes before I hit the "register" button on the race site. My running career up until that point included a bunch of short races, a single half-marathon, and intermittent training that rarely saw over-fifteen-mile weeks. On that fateful day that I dreamed I could run a marathon and then quickly threw money at the race directors, I had a little less than three months to prepare. I found a beginner's plan in a book at the library, made a photocopy, put the book with all its knowledge back on the shelf, and hurried off to try my first twenty-five-mile week ever.

This was dumb. I probably don't have to tell you that I spent many weeks aqua jogging the distances because shin splints made my legs feel like aliens were clawing through my bones. I felt exhausted the entire time I trained. I finished the race, but not without killer foot pain and great fatigue that plagued me for the next twelve months.

I know there are others like me, runners who bypass the earlier phases of marathon training to jump into the more intense weeks. Other marathoners add miles haphazardly. I'm here to tell you, not just from my own experience but from years of reporting on how the elite runners train, that proper marathon training is pivotal. Not only will a strong foundation help you avoid injury, it will give you a chance to get super strong before pushing your body to the limit.

DETERMINING WHERE YOU ARE IN YOUR RUNNING JOURNEY

Many training programs, plans, and apps lump runners into three categories: beginner, intermediate, advanced. Your training, though, is on a spectrum. Unless you are brand spanking new to running, you could shift and slide among all three of these categories depending on your goals, life outside of running, current fitness level, and emotional health. It's also essential to recognize that if you were once an advanced runner but maybe took a break, you might need to start at a slightly lower level. That doesn't mean you can't add "advanced" workouts to your routine when your body feels ready. All this is to say, I want you to pick a group and plan to follow, but I don't want you to feel locked in.

Many coaches and experts will base your level on previous race times and experience. But that might not be right for you. Let's break it down.

Beginner

You are new to running. You just ordered running shoes, and if I asked you how many miles you run per week, you might shrug. Maybe you've run a few blocks around town, but you don't know if that's five miles or half a mile. You're excited to embark on this process, but you're clueless. A newbie, a baby runner with so much to learn. You'll stay in this beginner phase until you are running three days or more per week and logging more than ten miles per week. You can also advance from beginner to intermediate when you run a 5K.

You might also be in the beginner category if

- your goal is to simply cross the finish line of a marathon;
- you are coming back from an injury or a long break;
- you have run a lot before, but your weekly mileage has dipped below ten miles per week;
- you've never run a marathon before; or
- you have never run before, period.

Intermediate

You have a few races under your belt and have crushed a 10K or half-marathon. If you are not currently training for your next race, then you are maintaining a fitness base. So when you think about your last week of running, it is likely that you ran a few days and the total mileage added up to more than ten and was actually closer to fifteen. If you're not quite up to ten weekly miles, consider yourself an advanced beginner, and follow the beginner plan to get your strength and endurance to where we want them to be.

Now let's talk goals. If you have run a marathon before and you are looking to run a PR, then yes, you are in the right place. But if your time goal is under 3:50, then move yourself to the advanced category.

You might also be an intermediate runner if

- you are aiming for a sub-4:30 marathon, at any age;
- you ran a half-marathon in less than two hours;
- you've never run a marathon before, but you train rigorously and can handle twenty or more miles per week with ease; or
- you've never run a marathon before, but you ran DII or DIII cross-country in college.

Advanced

When you get to the point when you're running thirty or more miles per week, you might be an advanced runner. You've run several races before, and you have finished at least one marathon at a speedy pace.

You might also be an advanced runner if

- you have run more than two marathons and finished in less than four hours;
- your goal is to qualify for Boston;
- you can't remember the last time you took a week off from running; or
- you've never run a marathon before, but you ran DI cross-country in college.

Beginner Training Cycle

If you're a new or beginner runner, I want you to consider a training cycle that is four parts: pre-base training, base training, in-season training, and maintenance. Each of these stages serves a different purpose. Each stage builds on the previous one to help you peak right around race time. The progressive build is to help your body handle the load without overexerting yourself.

Pre-base Training

5–10 months*
Build overall body strength, slow miles

---

* The length of pre-base depends on the individual runner. I'll outline it in more detail in the following sections.

Base Training

2 months

Build overall strength and begin increasing mileage, introduce medium-to-long runs

In-Season Training

4 months

Race-specific training, increase mileage and intensity, muscle maintenance

Maintenance

Beyond

After the race is over, easy workouts and cross-training

Intermediate and Advanced Training Cycle

If you're an intermediate or advanced runner, I recommend the cycle below.

Base Training

2 months

Build overall strength and begin increasing mileage, introduce medium-to-long runs

In-Season Training

4 months

Race-specific training, increase mileage and intensity, muscle maintenance

> ## Maintenance
>
> *Beyond*
> Easy workouts and cross-training

If it feels overwhelming right now, do not worry. The following pages will walk you through the process step by step. Each stage of marathoning will help you become a fitter, stronger, more determined version of yourself.

CHAPTER 3

CHOOSING THE RIGHT MARATHON

My recommendation is that you wait until your base training is nearly complete before registering for a marathon. In the training process, you'll discover your strengths and weaknesses, which will help you figure out what style of racecourse might be best for you.

However, since some marathon registration deadlines might fall before you complete your base training, I thought I would share some advice now on choosing the right marathon.

First—and this is critically important—make sure you'll have enough time to complete your training before the day of the marathon. If you're an intermediate or advanced runner, you'll want to make sure you have at least six months to train before the race. If you're a beginner, you should plan to have twelve to sixteen months to train before the race. (If you are a casual runner currently running fewer than ten miles a week, you'll want about twelve months to properly train. If you are completely new to running, you'll want about sixteen months to properly train.)

There are a plethora of marathons to choose from, and the good ones have their own identities. Grandma's Marathon in Duluth, Minnesota, is a weekend of festivities—a big race that attracts elites but still has a small-town feel. The Donna Marathon in Jacksonville, Florida, is a crusade for breast cancer research with survivors who run to celebrate life. There's Flying Pig in Cincinnati and Big Sur in Big Sur, California, and the St. George Marathon about three hours from where I live in Utah. Over the years, these races have become legendary. They are the gold standard of 26.2. You could race in so many amazing destinations or you could stay close to home. It's up to you, but you must choose wisely.

Picking the right race for your body, personality, and running style is really important. Now, I know that many beginners are probably thinking that the racecourse won't matter. Maybe you think you can just jump into your local marathon and be happy making to the finish. It helps, however, to think about how your strengths might match with a specific race to give you the best opportunity to enjoy the miles. For intermediate and advanced runners with aspirations of achieving a PR or qualifying for Boston, choosing the right race is imperative to your mission.

No matter who you are, here's what to think about.

WHEN IS THE RACE?

For many runners, choosing the right season to run in is the most important factor in picking a goal race. When thinking about running a fall race, consider that you'll be training during the summer months. Alternatively, if you choose a spring race, the bulk of your in-season will be during winter. If you live in a place with four seasons—or in a temperate climate with an extremely hot summer—you want to choose wisely to set yourself up for success.

In addition to factoring in temperatures during your race and training months, you have to look at your personal calendar and decide when you can devote the time to prepare and then race. In terms of the race weekend, think about whether you want to take a few days off from work before and after the big day (this might contribute to your decision about how far to travel away from home). I suggest you take at least one day off afterward, especially if it's a Sunday race. I made the mistake of returning to work the day following my first marathon, and I nearly wept walking up the stairs and then fell asleep in a meeting. Make the race your top priority for an entire week. Running for that long is stressful on your body, and when you finish, you deserve an incredible celebration.

HOW BIG IS THE MARATHON?

Some marathons, like the World Majors, are huge—thousands of runners and sometimes just as many spectators. Take, for example, the 2019 TCS New York City Marathon, which saw more than 53,000 finishers. That's a lot. There are advantages to this kind of race—the energy is spectacular, the crowds give you strength, and you're often running with (albeit far behind) elite runners. What other sport allows participants to compete (kind of) alongside Olympians? There are some other benefits too. Many of the bigger races boast courses that are designed to be speedy, so you'll encounter flatter routes and fewer turns. If you plan to use a pace group, the big races have experienced pacers and a big group to latch onto.

The downsides to these behemoth races? Welp, they are not for people who dread crowds. The logistics can be tiring. Finding your race packet, navigating the race expo, going through security, getting locked into your corral—this can add time on your feet in the hours before the race.

Luckily there are brilliant smaller races—some with fewer than eight hundred runners! Many of these will still be well organized and provide the same luxuries as their larger cousins (think: ample porta-potties and water stations).

WHERE IS THE RACE?

Many runners travel to make the whole ordeal a race-cation. Other runners choose a nearby race to avoid the stress of travel before the big day. You have to decide: Are you a runner who will embrace the added excitement? Or are you someone who needs a little more control of their environment? Here's the beginning of a pros list. I encourage you to make your own.

Destination race pros:

See a new place!
Add to the celebration
Eat at restaurants
Knock a race off your bucket list

Staying close to home pros:

Train on the actual racecourse
Sleep at home the night before
Eat at home
Routine and comfort

WHAT IS THE COURSE LIKE?

Now is the time to dial in and know your body. If you feel pretty comfortable judging what type of racecourse will help you make the most of your race, then turn your attention to those little maps on race websites.

There are some givens: a net downhill course will likely give you an advantage, as will a mostly straight race. (If you're trying to BQ, make sure the race is a qualifier.) Personal preferences will give you an edge when planning your race strategy.

Personally, I know that a pancake-flat course will hurt my body and mind. Having to create all my own momentum causes my bum hamstring to ache, my butt to fall asleep, and my brain to get incredibly bored. I look for racecourses that one might call "rolling." I like a lot of small hills—plenty of ascents and descents—so I check out the elevation maps to determine if the race will be good for me. If you hate hills, do not choose a rolling course!

Now, what about turns? You might not think they are a big deal, but turning costs valuable seconds and, for some people, will aggravate various tendons in the lower extremities. You can tell by the course map if the race is winding or if there are big straightaways where you will potentially turn your wheels.

DON'T FORGET THE DETAILS!

There are plenty of other nuances you might want to consider. Cost is a big one! Some of these races are very expensive. Compare a few before you throw all your dollars down. Does the method of timing matter to you? Do you need a race without a time limit so you can cross the finish at your leisure? What is the start time, and can you handle it? I mean, Disney races require you to be out of bed by 3:00 a.m., and for some, that is totally fine. But for me, that is a total deal breaker. Here's a comprehensive list of things that you might not think matter but will.

Organization

Being a race director is a really challenging job that requires a crazy amount attention to detail and the ability to manage a staff, sponsors, vendors, hundreds of porta-potties, and thousands of runners. I guarantee that you will not understand the value of race organization and knowledgeable staff until you run a sh*tshow of a race. The best races have an easy bib pickup, a method to their security, and directions to your starting corral (and starting corrals in general, for that matter; you do not want the start to be a free-for-all with six-hour marathoners lining up next to subthree folks). The premier races earn a reputation for being incredible, but there are definitely hidden gems all around. Ask locals about the race. If you are eyeing a race far from your home that doesn't have a lot of buzz around it, call the local running shop and ask some questions. You can start with "I'm thinking about running the marathon in your town. Can you tell me about it?" They will be happy to help or refer you to someone who can.

Security

Large marathons will have security, including metal detectors, bag searches, and a large police presence. These features were not as extreme before the Boston bombings. But now they are necessary, and the races do a really good job of ensuring our safety. If this kind of stuff makes you nervous, opt for a smaller race, but still ensure that there are some protective measures in place.

Medical Staff

Every race should have medical personnel on-site, and most will have the partnering doctors, hospital, or first responders listed in their race information.

Course Cutoff Time

My back-of-the-packers: There are some races that offer unlimited time or have generous time limits. If you aren't familiar with this concept, allow me to explain. Many races have to cap the time of finishers, not because they are mean but because cities need their streets reopened within six or seven hours. Sometimes there's a sweeper vehicle (like a van, bus, or golf cart) trailing behind the pack that's bringing up the rear. I've run in the back before at a race (the Donna Marathon) that allowed for a 6:30 completion. I needed to run slower for that marathon because I hadn't trained enough and needed to run-walk slowly to prevent injury. It was really nice knowing that I had a big time window to mosey along the course. If the race had had a six-hour cap, I would've felt a little bit rushed and stressed out. If you know you're going to need more time, find those races that let you do you.

Spectator Friendliness

You will have friends and family who want to see your smiling face out on the course! They have been watching you train, and they want to celebrate your accomplishment. Some races make it easy for crowds to see runners at multiple locations. If you want your support team out there at various miles, then plan for it and choose a marathon that offers easy-to-maneuver viewing. Even if your besties can't make it, crowd support is something to consider. Do you want strangers cheering you on for the majority of the race? Great! You can ask locals if the city or town gets into marathon morning. You can bet that the larger the race, the more fans will be out with signs, pom-poms, and cowbells!

If you're interested in a race but not sure about it after a decent amount of research, you can check out bibrave.com to see other runners' reviews.

Unfortunately, when it comes to race day, we can only control so much, even if we choose the absolute best race ever. Mother nature might bestow upon us a ninety-degree day with downpours. Even if we're sleeping in our own bed, we might toss and turn for a week before the race. We might lose our pace group, miss a water station, find a stray dog, cramp up unexpectedly. And you know what? None of that will be in the race descriptions.

What it ultimately comes down to is this: Does this race match my personal preferences? Will the course play to my strengths? Does it line up with my life? Most important, does it feel right?

CHAPTER 4

THE DYNAMIC WARM-UP

Before we do any running at all, we have to talk about prerun drills. I see way too many runners skip any kind of warm-up routine. They jet off and settle into their normal pace and probably don't realize how important it is to prime the body before the run.

For example, there is a syndrome that many female runners run into over the course of their training lives: sleeping-butt syndrome. It sounds ridiculous, but it's totally real. Basically, your gluteus medius and gluteus minimus muscles are very often ignored. Danielle Zickl, the health and fitness editor at *Runner's World*, says that this creates an imbalance: "Is your butt really asleep? No. But it's slacking off and that doesn't bode well for our form." Many of our bodies adapt and use the wrong areas to compensate while we're running. So instead of power coming from your booty, the forward momentum originates in your hip flexors or lower back. Strain in those places results in pain. The solution is to activate that butt before you run.

Before every run, do one circuit of the following moves. It might look like a lot, but it will take only five minutes total. Do each drill for about thirty seconds. Your heart rate should increase slightly, your body parts will feel more limber, and you will be amazed by how much easier your first mile will feel.

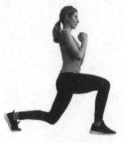

Walking Lunges with Twist

10 repetitions (5 on each leg, alternating)

This is a great move to fire up your glutes (booty) every time you run. Lunge forward with your right leg, keeping both knees bent ninety degrees. Squeeze your butt as you lunge, and twist your torso so that you are facing right (when you switch sides and lunge forward with your left leg, you'll twist to face left). Inhale, and return to standing. Switch legs.

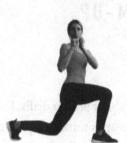

Windmill Tin Man Walks

10 repetitions on each leg, alternating

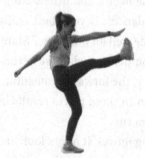

Complete this move to get your hamstrings, obliques, and shoulders going simultaneously. Start in an athletic stance. This is a term I will use a lot, so here's what that means: Stand with your feet shoulder width apart with a slight bend in your knees. Keep your chest lifted, back straight. Arms should be at your sides. To picture this, think about what a basketball player looks like just before the ball toss. Lift your right leg straight up in front of you until it is hip height and parallel to the ground. Simultaneously swing your left arm back, then around, and reach to your toes. Repeat on the other side.

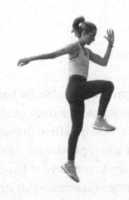

A-Skip

10 repetitions

Incredible for speed and power, this warm-up is used by athletes in many sports and is a favorite of four-time Olympian and winner of the Boston and New York marathons Meb Keflezighi. You might want to start slow and walk through it first to get the rhythm down. To begin, skip forward and lift your right knee up to waist height. Your left leg should remain straight as you launch off your toe. Swing your left arm, bent at ninety degrees, forward as your right knee comes up. Continue moving forward, skipping with the other leg and arm next. Keep your feet close together. Land on the balls of your feet.

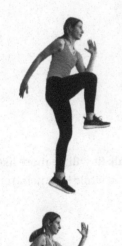

B-Skip

10 repetitions

The beginning of a B-skip is exactly the same as that of an A-skip. But when the knee is lifted, kick the bottom of the leg so that it extends straight out. Imagine making a lowercase *h* with your body that quickly turns into an uppercase *L*. Next, drop the raised leg so it lands slightly ahead of the back leg. Alternate using the same skipping motion as the A-skip.

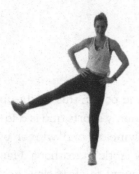

Side Leg Swings

10 repetitions on each side

If needed, hold on to something stable for balance, such as a tree or fence or sturdy chair. Swing your leg out to the side and then in front of you to the other side, like a pendulum. Keep your foot flexed. Don't try to reach your leg as high as it can go in either direction—you are simply looking to generate a little heat in your hips.

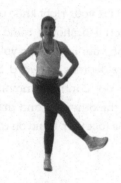

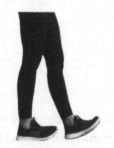

Walk on Your Heels

30 seconds

Lift your toes up and walk (it will be more like a waddle) in a straight line while balancing on your heels.

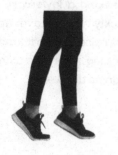

Walk on Your Toes

30 seconds

Lift your heels from the floor and balance on your toes. Walk in a straight line like you are wearing invisible high heels.

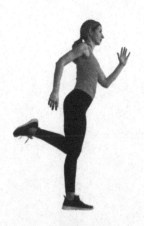

Butt Kicks

30 seconds

Start slow, marching at first, and bring your right heel to your butt, then your left. Slowly increase your speed. You should feel this mostly in your calves and a little bit in your quads.

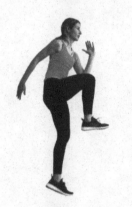

High Knees

30 seconds

Again, start slowly and accelerate as you go. Keeping your torso upright, drive your knees toward your chest, generating the power from your lower abs and glutes, and swing your arms forward and back.

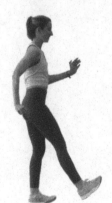

Straight Leg Bounds

30 seconds

Think of your legs like blades of scissors. With your torso upright, core tight, and legs straight, scissor-kick your way forward, bounding from alternating legs. The foot that is in the air should be flexed toward your knee (toes not pointed). You should land on the ball of your other foot.

This drill recruits your legs and hamstrings. If you feel you are using your hip flexors or lower back, stop and adjust.

PRE-BASE TRAINING

5-10 months

Goals: Build overall body strength, slow miles

If you're a new or beginner runner, the first training phase for you is pre-base (if you're an intermediate or advanced runner, you can skip this chapter and jump ahead to the next). Pre-base is a beautiful phase that cannot be ignored. When I first started running as an adult, I thought it would be totally fine if I ran one mile the first day, added a second mile on day two, and then forced myself to run four miles on day three. I did it and felt extraordinarily proud. On day four, I didn't want to get out of bed. Nothing in particular hurt, but I was dead tired. I know I probably ran too fast, and it didn't help that my lungs and liver and kidneys were still recovering from a number of hard-partying years that ultimately fueled my love of distance running. Anyway, what ended up happening was a lot of delayed-onset muscle soreness. I let a whole week go by before I ventured to run again. That's when I decided to consult the internet. The thing is, I wasn't necessarily totally new to running, but I'd taken five years off. Long breaks—even just months long—can put you back into beginner mode. What I'm trying to say is that you need to increase your running time slowly. That's what pre-base will help you do.

Pre-Base A

Week	Monday	Tuesday	Wednesday
1	•Walk 20 minutes	•Run-walk 15 minutes (walk 2 minutes, run 1 minute)	•Strength A + C (page 136 + 144)
2	•Walk 20 minutes	•Run-walk 15 minutes (walk 2 minutes, run 2 minutes)	•Strength A + C
3	•Strength A + C	•Run-walk 15 minutes (walk 2 minutes, run 3 minutes)	•Walk 30 minutes
4	•Strength A + C	•Run-walk 15 minutes (walk 5 minutes, run 5 minutes)	•Walk 30 minutes
5	•Strength A + C	•Run-walk 15 minutes (walk 5 minutes, run 5 minutes)	•Walk 30 minutes
6	•Strength A + C	•Run-walk 20 minutes (walk 5 minutes, run 10 minutes)	•Walk 30 minutes
7	•Strength A + C	•Run-walk 25 minutes (walk 5 minutes, run 10 minutes)	•Walk 30 minutes
8	•Strength A + C	•Run-walk 25 minutes (walk 5 minutes, run 10 minutes)	•Walk 30 minutes
9	•Rest	•Run-walk 30 minutes (walk 3 minutes, run 15 minutes)	•Rest
10	•Strength A + C •Walk 20 minutes	•Run-walk 30 minutes (walk 3 minutes, run 15 minutes)	•Walk 30 minutes
11	•Strength A + C •Walk 20 minutes	•Run-walk 25 minutes (walk 5 minutes, run 20 minutes)	•Walk 30 minutes
12	•Strength A + C •Walk 30 minutes	•Run-walk 20 minutes (walk 5 minutes, run 15 minutes)	•Walk 30 minutes
13	•Strength A + C •Walk 20 minutes	•Run-walk 20 minutes (walk 5 minutes, run 20 minutes)	•Walk 30 minutes
14	•Strength A + C •Walk 20 minutes	•Run-walk 31 minutes (walk 1 minute, run 30 minutes)	•Walk 30 minutes
15	•Strength A + C •Walk 30 minutes	•Run-walk 31 minutes (walk 1 minute, run 30 minutes)	•Walk 30 minutes
16	•Strength A + C •Walk 30 minutes	•Run-walk 30 minutes (walk 1 minute, run 30 minutes)	•Rest

Thursday	Friday	Saturday	Sunday
•Rest	•Run-walk 15 minutes (walk 2 minutes, run 1 minute)	•Run-walk 30 minutes (walk 2 minutes, run 1 minute)	•Rest
•Rest	•Run-walk 20 minutes (walk 2 minutes, run 2 minutes)	•Run-walk 30 minutes (walk 2 minutes, run 2 minutes)	•Rest
•Run-walk 25 minutes (walk 2 minutes, run 3 minutes)	•Rest	•Run-walk 30 minutes (walk 2 minutes, run 3 minutes)	•Rest
•Run-walk 30 minutes (walk 5 minutes, run 5 minutes)	•Rest	•Run-walk 30 minutes (walk 5 minutes, run 5 minutes)	•Rest
•Run-walk 25 minutes (walk for 5 minutes, run 5 minutes)	•Rest	•Run-walk 30 minutes (walk 5 minutes, run 5 minutes)	•Rest
•Run-walk 25 minutes (walk 5 minutes, run 10 minutes)	•Rest	•Run-walk 30 minutes (walk 5 minutes, run 10 minutes)	•Rest
•Run-walk 25 minutes (walk 5 minutes, run 10 minutes)	•Rest	•Run-walk 30 minutes walk 5 minutes, run 10 minutes)	•Rest
•Run-walk 30 minutes (walk 5 minutes, run 10 minutes)	•Rest	•Run a 5K race!*	•Walk 20 minutes
•Run-walk 30 minutes (walk 3 minutes, run 15 minutes)	•Rest	•Run-walk 35 minutes (walk 3 minutes, run 15 minutes)	•Rest
•Run-walk 25 minutes (walk 3 minutes, run 15 minutes)	•Rest	•Run-walk 35 minutes (walk 3 minutes, run 15 minutes)	•Rest
•Run-walk 25 minutes (walk 5 minutes, run 20 minutes)	•Rest	•Run-walk 35 minutes (walk 5 minutes, run 20 minutes)	•Rest
•Run-walk 15 minutes (walk 5 minutes, run 10 minutes)	•Rest	•Run-walk 40 minutes (walk 5 minutes, run 25 minutes)	•Rest
•Run-walk 25 minutes (walk 5 minutes, run 20 minutes)	•Rest	•Run-walk 40 minutes (walk 5 minutes, run 30 minutes)	•Rest
•Run-walk 21 minutes (walk 1 minute, run 20 minutes)	•Rest	•Run-walk 45 minutes (walk 1 minute, run 30 minutes)	•Rest
•Run-walk 25 minutes (walk 1 minute, run 24 minutes)	•Rest	•Run-walk 45 minutes (walk 1 minute, run 30 minutes)	•Rest
•Run-walk 30 minutes (walk 1 minute, run 30 minutes)	•Rest	•Run-walk 45 minutes (walk 1 minute, run 30 minutes)	•Rest

* If you decide not to run a 5K, try running a 3.1-mile time trial instead.

If you've got your sights set on running a marathon, it is incredibly important that you get time on your feet without exhausting yourself. If you've never run or if you're currently running fewer than ten miles per week, it is essential to play it safe. Start with this pre-base kick-start program to safely increase your running volume.

Because pre-base is for people ramping up from little to no running, every run should be slow and easy. Many of the first runs are run-walk, meaning they alternate between walking and running in time intervals. If the plan says "Run-walk 30 minutes (walk for three minutes, run for fifteen minutes)," then

Pre-Base B

Week	Monday	Tuesday	Wednesday
1	•Walk 20 minutes	•Run 15 minutes	•Strength A + C (page 136 + 144)
2	•Walk 20 minutes	•Run 15 minutes	•Strength A + C
3	•Strength A + C	•Run 15 minutes	•Walk 30 minutes
4	•Strength A + C	•Run 15 minutes	•Walk 30 minutes
5	•Strength A + C	•Run 15 minutes	•Walk 30 minutes
6	•Strength A + C	•Run 20 minutes	•Walk 30 minutes
7	•Strength A + C	•Run 25 minutes	•Walk 30 minutes
8	•Strength A + C	•Run 25 minutes	•Walk 30 minutes
9	•Rest	•Run 30 minutes	•Rest
10	•Strength A + C •Walk 20 minutes	•Run 30 minutes	•Walk 30 minutes
11	•Strength A + C •Walk 20 minutes	•Run 25 minutes	•Walk 30 minutes
12	•Strength A + C •Walk 30 minutes	•Run 20 minutes	•Walk 30 minutes
13	•Strength A + C •Walk 20 minutes	•Run 20 minutes	•Walk 30 minutes

follow that pattern of walking for three minutes and running for fifteen minutes until the thirty minutes are up. Don't worry if your time is up in the middle of a run. Just follow the pattern, get to the allotted time, and celebrate when you finish.

In week 8, you have the option of running a 5K race. Keep it nice and easy, but enjoy the excitement.

If you're starting from zero running ever, see Pre-base A.

If you're a casual runner currently running fewer than ten miles a week, see Pre-base B.

Thursday	Friday	Saturday	Sunday
•Rest	•Run 15 minutes	•Run 30 minutes	•Rest
•Rest	•Run 20 minutes	•Run 30 minutes	•Rest
•Run 25 minutes	•Rest	•Run 30 minutes	•Rest
•Run 30 minutes	•Rest	•Run 30 minutes	•Rest
•Run 25 minutes	•Rest	•Run 30 minutes	•Rest
•Run 25 minutes	•Rest	•Run 30 minutes	•Rest
•Run 25 minutes	•Rest	•Run 30 minutes	•Rest
•Run 30 minutes	•Rest	•Run a 5K race!*	•Walk 20 minutes
•Run 30 minutes	•Rest	•Run 35 minutes	•Rest
•Run 25 minutes	•Rest	•Run 35 minutes	•Rest
•Run 25 minutes	•Rest	•Run 35 minutes	•Rest
•Run 15 minutes	•Rest	•Run 40 minutes	•Rest
•Run 25 minutes	•Rest	•Run 40 minutes	•Rest

* If you decide not to run a 5K, try running a 3.1-mile time trial instead.

Week	Monday	Tuesday	Wednesday
14	•Strength A + C •Walk 20 minutes	•Run 30 minutes	•Walk 30 minutes
15	•Strength A + C •Walk 30 minutes	•Run 30 minutes	•Walk 30 minutes
16	•Strength A + C •Walk 30 minutes	•Run 30 minutes	•Rest
17	•Strength A + C •Walk 30 minutes	•Run 35 minutes	•Rest
18	•Strength A + C •Walk 30 minutes	•Run 35 minutes	•Rest
19	•Strength A + C •Walk 30 minutes	•Run 30 minutes	•Rest
20	•Strength A + C •Walk 30 minutes	•Run 30 minutes	•Rest
21	•Strength A + C •Walk 30 minutes	•Run 30 minutes	•Rest
22	•Strength A + C •Walk 30 minutes	•Run 30 minutes	•Rest

A FEW NOTES ABOUT PLANS

I may repeat this phrase a few times: do not feel like you have to adhere to the plan at all costs. There will be days that you can't get your miles in because you have to work late. Or your family needs you. Or all your sports bras are in the laundry and they smell too bad to rewear (been there).

Later in the book, when we get to in-season plans, I'll tell you not to make up miles when you miss them. But right now, because a good portion of the time spent on your feet is walking, it is acceptable to do the workout you missed the next day. If you miss a day and you don't have time to make it up, that is absolutely, totally fine. Just move on.

In the plans, you'll notice a 5K race or 3.1-mile time trial listed on a Saturday. If you choose to do a road race, you might sign up for a race that's on a

Thursday	Friday	Saturday	Sunday
·Run 20 minutes	·Rest	·Run 45 minutes	·Rest
·Run 25 minutes	·Rest	·Run 45 minutes	·Rest
·Run 30 minutes	·Rest	·Run 45 minutes	·Rest
·Run 30 minutes	·Rest	·Run 50 minutes	·Rest
·Run 30 minutes	·Rest	·Run 50 minutes	·Rest
·Run 30 minutes	·Rest	·Run 50 minutes	·Rest
·Run 30 minutes	·Rest	·Run 55 minutes	·Rest
·Run 30 minutes	·Rest	·Run 55 minutes	·Rest
·Run 30 minutes	·Rest	·Run 55 minutes	·Rest

Sunday. No sweat—rest on Saturday, race on Sunday, do a twenty-minute walk on the Monday following the race, then pick up the plan from there.

WHEN TO MOVE ON

For my newbies starting with no running experience, I advise going through both pre-base plans. The run-walk plan (pre-base A) will gradually get you into running shape. When you complete it, which takes four months, then jump on over to pre-base B.

I can hear some of you asking: "What if I want to skip a few weeks? What if I'm sick of run-walking?" Yeah, that very well might happen. You'll also notice that if you are sticking to the plan, your fitness will skyrocket. If you get to the start of week 12 of pre-base A, and you realize that you can handle twenty-five minutes of running with relative ease (meaning your breathing is relaxed, you can maintain an easy pace, your legs feel great) then I want you to try running thirty minutes straight on that Saturday instead of the recommended twenty-five. Keep your walking intervals the same length. At the end of that run, be honest with yourself. If it was easy-peasy, it's time to start following the pre-base B plan—starting from the beginning.

Pre-base B is intended to work you up to about twelve miles per week, as long as you're running a pace of twelve minutes per mile or less. If you're running slower, it's OK, because you're still getting the right amount of time on your feet. Once you get to the end of pre-base B, you can move to the base plan.

I want to tell you something about these plans: they are *very* conservative. They are built to ensure you get to in-season training, and ultimately the marathon, injury free. So if you are starting from *zero* or close to zero, this process will take quite some time and patience. That patience is self-love. It's giving yourself the time and space to be the very best you can be. It's understanding that you need to start where you are. If that's absolutely no miles and a brand-new pair of running shoes, then think about the thrilling journey that is in front of you. Yeah, it might take twelve or sixteen months to reach the finish line. Decide right now if your *why* is worth the commitment. If you're still reading, then I know you're determined. I know you're ready.

CHAPTER 6

BASE TRAINING

2 months

Goals: Build overall strength and begin increasing mileage, introduce medium-to-long runs

uilding your base is serious business! Think of your pre-base as your foundation, like you poured some concrete in a hole in the ground. This next phase, the base phase, is the framework. Unless you want your marathon house to collapse as you hang the drywall, you need to construct the next eight weeks with care.

Base training is a lot of work. Our base is where we figure out what's working and what's not working. It's where we increase our mileage, build muscle, and perform a variety of physical tests to understand our strengths and weaknesses. In this program, you'll also start a process of self-discovery.

Here is what your base training plan will look like. If you're a beginner, this plan might not make much sense right now (for example, what's a VO2 max test?). I'll explain it all in the pages to come.

Beginner Base Training Plan

Week	Monday	Tuesday	Wednesday	Thursday	Friday	Saturday	Sunday
1	•Strength test (page 43)	•Easy run 30 minutes	•Walk 20 minutes	•Magic Mile test (page 61)	•Rest/walk	•Long run 50 minutes	•Rest/walk
2	•Strength D (page 48)	•Easy run 30 minutes	•Walk 20 minutes •Strength E (page 53)	•Easy run 25 minutes	•Rest/walk	•Long run 55 minutes	•Rest/walk
3	•Strength D	•Easy run 30 minutes	•Walk 20 minutes •Strength E	•Easy run 25 minutes	•Rest/walk	•Long run 55 minutes	•Rest/walk
4	•Strength D	•Easy run 30 minutes	•Intervals test (page 79) •Strength E	•Easy run 30 minutes	•Rest/walk	•Long run 60 minutes	•Rest/walk
5	•Strength D •Cross-train 30 minutes (page 58)	•Easy run 20 minutes	•Repeats test (page 81) •Strength E	•Easy run 20 minutes	•Rest/walk	•Long run 55 minutes	•Rest/walk
6	•Strength D •Cross-train 30 minutes	•Easy run 30 minutes	•Hill test (page 82) •Strength E	•Easy run 20 minutes	•Rest/walk	•Long run 65 minutes	•Rest/walk
7	•Strength D •Cross-train 30 minutes	•Easy run 30 minutes	•Tempo test (page 85) •Strength E	•Easy run 25 minutes	•Rest/walk	•Long run 60 minutes	•Rest/walk
8	•Strength D •Cross-train 30 minutes	•Easy run 35 minutes	•VO2 max test (page 87) •Strength E	•Easy run 30 minutes	•Rest/walk	•Long run 70 minutes	•Rest/walk

Intermediate Base Training Plan

Week	Monday	Tuesday	Wednesday	Thursday	Friday	Saturday	Sunday
1	•Strength Test (page 43)	•Easy run 3 miles	•Walk 20 minutes •Strength E (page 53)	•Magic Mile Test (page 61) •Easy run 2 miles	•Rest/ walk	•Long run 6 miles	•Rest/walk
2	•Strength D (page 48)	•Easy run 3.5 miles	•Walk 20 minutes •Strength E	•Easy run 3.5 miles	•Rest/ walk	•Long run 7 miles	•Rest/walk
3	•Strength D	•Easy run 5 miles	•Walk 20 minutes •Strength E	•Easy run 3 miles	•Rest/ walk	•Long run 7 miles	•Rest/walk
4	•Strength D	•Easy run 4 miles	•Intervals Test (page 79) •Strength E	•Easy run 4 miles	•Rest/ walk	•Long run 7 miles	•Rest/walk
5	•Strength D •Cross-train 30 minutes (page 58)	•Easy run 5 miles	•Repeats Test (page 81) •Strength E	•Easy run 3 miles	•Rest/ walk	•Long run 6.5 miles	•Rest/walk
6	•Strength D •Cross-train 30 minutes	•Easy run 5 miles	•Hill Test (page 82) •Strength E	•Easy run 3 miles	•Rest/ walk	•Long run 7 miles	•Rest/walk
7	•Strength D •Cross-train 30 minutes	•Easy run 4 miles	•Tempo Test (page 85) •Strength E	•Easy run 3.5 miles	•Rest/ walk	•Long run 8 miles	•Rest/walk
8	•Strength D •Cross-train 30 minutes	•Easy run 2.5 miles	•VO2 Max Test (page 87) •Strength E	•Easy run 3 miles	•Rest/ walk	•Long run 7 miles	•Rest/walk

Advanced Base Training Plan

Week	Monday	Tuesday	Wednesday	Thursday	Friday	Saturday	Sunday
1	•Strength Test (page 43)	•Easy run 4 miles	•Easy run 3 miles	•Magic Mile Test (page 61) •Easy run 2 miles	•Rest/ walk	•Long run 6 miles	•Rest/walk
2	•Strength D (page 48) •Cross-train 30 minutes (page 58)	•Easy run 4 miles	•Easy run 3 miles •Strength E (page 53)	•Easy run 3 miles	•Rest/ walk	•Long run 7 miles	•Rest/walk
3	•Strength D •Cross-train 30 minutes	•Easy run 5 miles	•Easy run 3 miles •Strength E	•Easy run 3 miles	•Rest/ walk	•Long run 7 miles	•Rest/walk
4	•Strength D •Cross-train 30 minutes	•Easy run 4 miles	•Intervals Test (page 79) •Strength E	•Easy run 3 miles	•Rest/ walk	•Long run 6 miles	•Rest/walk
5	•Strength D •Cross-train 30 minutes	•Easy run 5 miles	•Repeats Test (page 81) •Easy run 2 miles •Strength E	•Easy run 3 miles	•Rest/ walk	•Long run 6.5 miles	•Rest/walk
6	•Strength D •Cross-train 30 minutes	•Easy run 5 miles	•Hill Test (page 82) •Easy run 3 miles •Strength E	•Easy run 3 miles	•Rest/ walk	•Easy run 7 miles	•Rest/walk
7	•Strength D •Cross-train 30 minutes	•Easy run 5 miles	•Tempo Test (page 85) •Easy run 3 miles •Strength E	•Easy run 3.5 miles	•Rest/ walk	•Long run 8 miles	•Rest/walk
8	•Strength D •Cross-train 30 minutes	•Easy run 2.5 miles	•VO2 Max Test (page 87) •Strength E	•Easy run 3 miles	•Rest/ walk	•Long run 7 miles	•Rest/walk

WHY START WITH STRENGTH?

The first thing you'll see on the base training plan is "strength test." Why start with strength? Let me explain with this tale of warning. I have a dear friend who is a superb runner. Her name is Emily and her marathon PR is 3:01. Pretty speedy, right? We once visited my trainer together—a man who prides himself on injury prevention and building lean muscle mass. He asked us to do step-ups onto a twenty-inch box. That's all. Just step up onto the box with one foot, bring the other foot up, then step back down.

Emily wobbled. She fell over sideways off the box like a baby deer taking its first steps. The trainer asked what strength work she'd put in throughout her five-year-long marathon career. None. Then he asked her how many times she'd been injured. Five.

The problem, he explained, was that the muscles in Emily's body had grown so accustomed to propelling her forward that the lateral movement and core muscles, which keep you stabilized and balanced, had basically fallen asleep. You might think that's OK for runners, but it's not. Deficiencies in functional movements and overuse of certain muscle groups will inevitably cause injury.

The bottom line? You want to build some muscle here, people. (Not too much, because we don't want too much bulk.) Timing is important. You need to put in the work now, during base training, so that you can just maintain during the in-season training period. Now is also the time to add some plyometrics. It's been proven that explosive movements like jumping and hopping recruit your fast-twitch muscles and add speed, even for endurance athletes. These moves place tension and strain on our muscles and joints, so it's better to put them in play during the base phase, when your mileage is still low. We take them out during in-season training.

Strength Test

Do you have deficits that could impact your speed or lead to injury? Complete the following exercises with or without weights. If you have a mirror or camera available, use it to get the complete picture of how your body responds to the following moves.

Split Squat

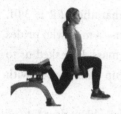

10 repetitions on each leg

Stand with your right foot forward and your left foot propped on a chair or bench behind you. Bend your right knee so that it descends slowly into a lunge position—end with your right leg at ninety degrees. Complete a rep by returning to the starting position. Do all ten reps on one side. Then switch so that your left leg is in front and your right leg is propped up behind you.

What to watch out for: Your knees. If you do not have adequate strength in your quadriceps and hips, your front knee may collapse inward (it should be pointing slightly out away from your body). If you have balance issues in this position, poor ankle flexibility could be the culprit. Your chest should remain upright.

Why: Split squats will test the stability and mobility of your foot, ankle, knee, and hip. Practicing this move with perfect form will improve the strength and movement of all the above.

Were split squats challenging?

_____

_____

Did you notice any issues?

_____

_____

Single-Leg Dead Lift

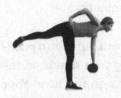

10 repetitions per leg (complete on right side first, then switch to the left side)

Stand on your right leg. Keeping your right knee slightly bent, perform a stiff-legged dead lift by bending at the hip while extending your left leg behind you for balance. Continue bending forward until you are parallel to the ground, and then return to the upright position. Complete all ten repetitions on one side, then repeat on the other side. If this move is too simple, grab a dumbbell and complete the move with the weight in the hand opposite the leg that is in the air.

What to watch for: Balance issues, shaking, collapsing on one side. Forcing the body to maintain stability on one leg will help show imbalances between the left and right sides.

Why: The single-leg dead lift not only develops hip strength and power but also allows the muscles of the hips and legs to act as stabilizers.

How was your single-leg dead lift form overall?

_____

_____

Did one side differ from the other?

_____

_____

Low Plank

Time yourself for up to 2 minutes

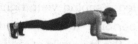

Position yourself like you're about to do a push-up, but instead of placing your hands on the floor, place your forearms on the floor. Your elbows should be below your shoulders. You can place your palms flat on the ground or clasp your hands together. Your feet should be apart, in line with your shoulders. Engage your core, squeezing the muscles in your abs and glutes so that they stabilize your whole body. Ground the toes into the floor. Hold.

What to watch for: If your butt is too far up, you're making the move easier by taking tension out of your core. If your midsection begins to sag during the exercise, this indicates core weakness and will put pressure on your lower back. Your aim is to be strong enough to maintain proper form for at least two minutes.

Why: Trunk stability for runners is essential for good running posture. This will prevent a multitude of issues, including hip, glute, and IT band injuries.

Time: _____

How was your low plank?

_____

_____

Bird Dog

10 repetitions on each side

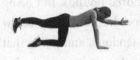

Get on all fours and extend your left arm and right leg at the same time, ensuring that they are parallel to the ground. Now bring both the left elbow and the right knee back underneath your body, so that they touch in the center. Return the arm and leg to the extended position. Then get back on all fours. Do the same thing on the other side.

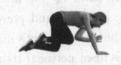

What to watch for: If there is weakness in the core, you may rotate your hips excessively. Wobbling or leaning too far to one side are other red flags.

Why: Rotational stability is another form of core strength and is essential for preventing back injuries in runners.

How were the bird dogs?

_____

_____

Heck yes! Good work completing the test. Some of this stuff isn't easy. Don't be sad if your body is not as strong as you want it to be. The only way to get better is to know your limitations and weaknesses. The program below is intended to help you do just that as you increase your mileage. But if you are noticing some imbalances, or if you noticed that some of the moves above felt very challenging, I want you to add them to the base training strength plan. Tack them on at the end of each strength circuit and take note when they start to feel easier.

The Base Training Strength Circuit

In running, no one cares if you can bench two hundred pounds. But being able to do ten good push-ups will increase your speed. The routine below is designed to keep the limbs, muscles, ligaments, tendons, and joints that we use for running happy and healthy. It shouldn't tax you so much that you're sore for the next run. However, it does include plyometric moves and more advanced exercises than what you'll see when you are in-season training. That's because now is the time to really build up the muscle groups that will increase your speed (thank you, jumping) and prevent injury (yes, that means lots of work to keep your butt awake). Let's make this circuit, designed by Daniel Moody, a CSCS-certified personal trainer who specializes in injury prevention and rehabilitation, a habit during the base months:

STRENGTH D

Go through this circuit three times:

Reverse Lunges

15 repetitions on each leg

Start by standing with your feet shoulder width apart and your hands behind your head. Your elbows should be bent, your palms resting flat against your head. Then take a large, controlled step backward with your right foot. Lower yourself so that your left leg is bent at a ninety-degree angle and your left thigh is parallel to the ground. Make sure your left knee is directly above your left ankle. Your right leg should also be bent at a ninety-degree angle. Your right shin should be parallel to the ground, and your right knee should be in line with your right ankle. Return to standing for one rep. Maintain your hand position for the entirety of the set. Do fifteen reps on one leg, then switch to the other leg.

Side Lunges

15 repetitions on each leg

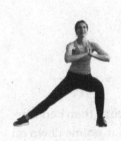

Start by standing with your feet shoulder width apart and your hands on your hips. Keep your shoulders back and down, your head up, and your core stable. Keeping an upright posture, step your right leg out to the right side. Your right foot should land parallel to your left foot, with your right knee bent at ninety degrees. Your left leg should be straight. Keep your feet pointed straight ahead. In stepping out, your body will shift to the right slightly and your weight will be placed on the right leg. Return to standing for one rep. Do fifteen reps on one side and then switch to the other leg.

Dumbbell Dead Lift

10 repetitions

Choose dumbbells that are challenging but not so heavy that you have to put them down

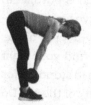

in the middle of a set. Starting with a set of five-pound weights and working up to fifteen pounds should be adequate for most runners. Holding the dumbbells at your sides, stand with your legs shoulder width apart, with a slight bend in the knees. Hinge at your hips so that your legs stay where they are but your upper body (above your hips) leans forward. Your back should remain straight. Bend your knees slightly, lowering the dumbbells to your shins without allowing your back to round. Brace your core. You should feel the tension in your hamstrings, glutes, and core muscles. Return to standing for one rep.

Inchworms

15 repetitions

Start by standing with your feet hip distance apart, then bend forward at your hips into a forward fold. Place your palms down on the ground, then walk your hands (in a million tiny steps, like you're an adorable tiny worm) forward into high plank. High plank is like the starting position for a push-up. Your hands should be under your shoulders, your feet still hip distance apart. Then walk your feet to meet your hands so that you're back in a forward fold. Stand up and repeat.

Squat with Dumbbell Overhead Press

15 repetitions

Stand with your feet shoulder width apart and your dumbbells in your hands, curled up

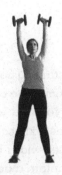

in front of your shoulders. Lower into a squat. In your squat, focus on keeping your chest up, your weight in your heels, your knees behind your toes, and your thighs turned out, meaning your knees should not collapse inward. From the squat, explode to standing and reach your dumbbells overhead. When you think of exploding, I want you to think of driving your hips forward to straighten your legs and using the momentum from your hips to propel the weight overhead. As you lift, rotate your arms so that your palms face away from you.

Single-Leg Hops

20 repetitions on each leg

Stand with your feet hip distance apart. Load your weight onto your right leg and foot, drawing your left knee up toward your chest. Jump on your right leg. Continue to hop twenty times on the same leg. Switch legs and repeat.

Push-ups

10 repetitions

You know how to do a push-up. Go for it!

High Plank

Hold for one minute

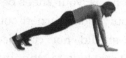

The high plank looks like the starting position for a push-up. Your palms should be on the floor and arms underneath you and in line with your shoulders. Your feet, knees, and quadriceps should be shoulder width apart and lifted off the ground. Maintain a neutral spine, meaning do not allow your butt to peak into the air or your hips to sag down toward the ground. Engage your core muscles (abs, back, and butt) to keep your body stable. Hold this position for one minute.

Low Plank

Hold for one minute

This is similar to high plank, except that your forearms are on the floor. Position yourself like you're about to do a push-up, but instead of placing your palms on the floor, place your forearms on the floor. Your elbows should be below your shoulders. You can place your palms flat on the ground or clasp your hands together. Your feet should be apart, in line with your shoulders. Engage your core, squeezing the muscles in your abs and glutes so that they stabilize your whole body. Ground the toes into the floor. Hold for one minute.

Low Side Plank

Hold for 30 seconds on each side

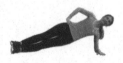

For this plank variation, start on your side, with your feet together and your right elbow directly below your shoulder. Raise your hips so that your body is in a straight line from head to feet. Place your left hand on your hip. Your right forearm and feet should be the only parts of your body touching the ground. Hold this position for thirty seconds. Switch sides and repeat. You should feel this in your obliques, which are the muscles on the sides of your abs. These do wonders for helping you maintain stability in your core while running.

STRENGTH E

Go through this circuit three times:

Jumping Jacks

30 repetitions

Remember these from PE? Yup, go for it.

Stationary Long Jump

5 repetitions

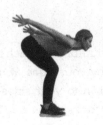

Start in a standing position with feet shoulder width apart and legs generously bent at the knees. You are going to jump forward from this position, using momentum from your arm swing. To achieve a great distance, start by swinging both arms behind you, keeping your elbows bent slightly. Then swing your arms forward and simultaneously jump straight ahead. In addition to the arm swing, you should use power from your legs, glutes, and hips to gain ground. Land softly on the balls of your feet with your knees slightly bent (both feet should touch the ground at the same time). Turn around and jump back to where you started. That's one rep.

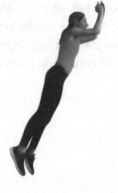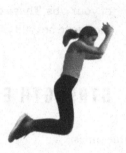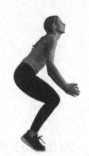

Prisoner Squats

15 repetitions

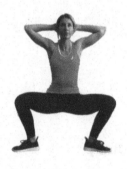

Start by standing with your feet slightly wider than shoulder width apart. With your hands behind your head and chest up, lower into a squat. Hold for a beat and return to standing.

Biceps Curls

15 repetitions

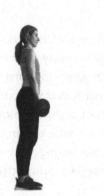

While standing, hold a dumbbell in each hand with your arms down by your sides. Your elbows should be tucked in to your sides and your palms should be facing forward. Then curl your forearms up while keeping your

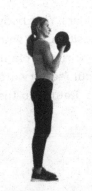

upper arms stationary. You want to bring the weights up to shoulder level. Return your arms to the starting position. If doing bicep curls on both arms at the same time is too challenging, you can alternate one arm at a time.

Triceps Dips

15 repetitions

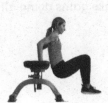

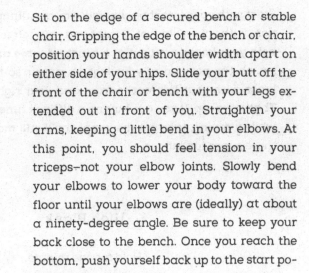

Sit on the edge of a secured bench or stable chair. Gripping the edge of the bench or chair, position your hands shoulder width apart on either side of your hips. Slide your butt off the front of the chair or bench with your legs extended out in front of you. Straighten your arms, keeping a little bend in your elbows. At this point, you should feel tension in your triceps—not your elbow joints. Slowly bend your elbows to lower your body toward the floor until your elbows are (ideally) at about a ninety-degree angle. Be sure to keep your back close to the bench. Once you reach the bottom, push yourself back up to the start position and repeat.

In-and-Outs

10 repetitions

These are just good old-fashioned fitness fun! Stand with your feet shoulder width apart and your arms by your sides. Lower into a squat position. Bend forward all the way until your hands are touching the floor and directly beneath your shoulders. Your body should look like you are in downward-facing dog position, but with very bent knees. From here, kick or step your legs back into a plank position. Then engage your core to jump (or step) your feet forward to starting position. Then rise back into a squat. Return to the standing position.

Jumping Lunges

10 repetitions

Start with your feet shoulder width apart. Jump into a lunge position, with your right foot in front and your left foot back. Make sure both your knees are bent at a ninety-degree angle. Jump up and switch the position of your legs in midair so that you land in a lunge with your left foot in front and your right foot behind you. That's one rep. If you are having a difficult time maintaining form while jumping, take out the jump! You'll still make gains doing all these super fun lunges.

High Plank

Hold for one minute

The high plank looks like the starting position for a push-up. Your palms should be on the floor and arms underneath you and in line with your shoulders. Your feet, knees, and quadriceps should be shoulder width apart and lifted off the ground. Maintain a neutral spine, meaning do not allow your butt to peak into the air or your hips to sag down toward the ground. Engage your core muscles (abs, back, and butt) to keep your body stable. Hold this position for one minute.

Low Plank

Hold for one minute

This is similar to high plank, except that your forearms are on the floor. Position yourself like you're about to do a push-up, but instead of placing your palms on the floor, place your forearms on the floor. Your elbows should be below your shoulders. You can place your palms flat on the ground or clasp your hands together. Your feet should be apart, in line with your shoulders. Engage your core, squeezing the muscles in your abs and glutes so that they stabilize your whole body. Ground the toes into the floor. Hold for one minute.

Low Side Plank

Hold for 30 seconds on each side

For this plank variation, start on your side, with your feet together and your right elbow directly below your shoulder. Raise your hips so that your body is in a straight line from head to feet. Place your left hand on your hip. Your right forearm and feet should be the only parts of your body touching the ground. Hold this position for thirty seconds. Switch sides and repeat. You should feel this in your obliques, which are the muscles on the sides of your abs. These do wonders for helping you maintain stability in your core while running.

CROSS-TRAINING

Cross-training is any cardio activity that isn't running. Maybe you're thinking, "Why would I need to do additional cardio that isn't running if I am running a marathon?" Varying your cardio is a useful tool in avoiding overuse injuries and preventing any running-specific training problems. The key is getting your heart rate up while your body is doing something different. This can help with muscle balance and strength while giving your brain a running break. Here are some ideas—feel free to experiment with different cross-training options.

Cross-Training Options for Marathoners

Swimming	Ice-skating
Road cycling	Rowing
Mountain biking	Stationary bike
Hiking	Elliptical

BUILDING MILEAGE

The base training period is when you'll start to train your body to run longer. One of the classic approaches for building mileage is the 10 percent rule. It's a really simple calculation: you take the number of miles you ran in the last week and increase it by 10 percent, and that's how many miles you run the following week. It's a gentle progression that's been around since at least the 1970s. The idea is that the slow progression will decrease the risk of injury from overuse.

I believe there are more effective ways to increase your aerobic endurance, time on your feet, and anaerobic tolerance simultaneously. Your mileage buildup does not need to be linear. The method I suggest mixes the 10 percent rule with step-down weeks, which are weeks that give your body a break by assigning fewer miles. The base training plan I shared earlier is based on this method.

New Jersey–based exercise scientist and RRCA-certified running coach Erica Coviello says: "What I find beneficial in my own training and that of most of my athletes is to bump up the long runs each week for three to four weeks, followed by a recovery week."

In the base plans, you'll see that all runners will have a decrease in the number of miles assigned in week 5. You still have a long run, but it's not as long.

Don't be surprised if those miles in week 5 feel tough even though you're running fewer miles than you were earlier. That's because you've spent the past month building strength, muscle, and endurance. That recovery week is a chance for your body to catch up.

Pace Yourself

Runners talk about pace so much. What is our race pace? What is our mile pace? What is our 5K pace? What is a "good" pace? Your pace is the time per mile that you run when completing a certain distance.

For example, if I ran a 20:10 5K, my pace per mile would be 6:29 per mile, meaning I would have run 3.1 miles at an average pace of 6:29 per mile. That's pretty fast, by the way.

Throughout your training, you will need to know the following paces:

- Easy-run pace: Your pace during your weekday casual miles.
- Long-run pace: Your pace during your weekend miles, exceeding fifty minutes. This will be the same as or even slower than your easy run pace.
- Speed-work paces: *Speed work* is a catchall phrase that refers to the various types of anaerobic training that runners use to get faster. Later in this chapter, I'll explain the different tests of speed that are in the base training plan (intervals test, repeats test, tempo test, etc.). We need to figure out what pace to run for each of these.
- Race pace: The average time per mile you run a given race distance (e.g., your 5K pace, your 10K pace, your marathon pace).

In the next section, I'll show you how to calculate paces.

But before you start calculating your paces, I want to emphasize something: the most important thing for you to know during base training is that every run during base training should be run at an easy pace except for the designated hard days (i.e., the days when you see a tempo test, intervals test, etc.).

The legendary coach Jenny Hadfield, who wrote a column for *Runner's World* and virtually trained probably thousands of people for marathons, says that long runs and easy runs are not about reaching a pace. They are about effort. So your pace might fluctuate on these runs based on a host of factors, including heat, stress, humidity, sleep, and nutrition.

That being said, I want you to look at your easy- and long-run training paces, because I'm nearly 100 percent certain that you're running them too dang fast. These "easy" paces should sometimes be torturous, because they are meant to be run very slowly.

Calculating Paces

In your first week of base training, a few days after your strength test, you'll have a one-mile time trial. You might think that a one-mile time would be frivolous in any race longer than a 5K, but it can actually provide you with important data.

The Magic Mile Test

- Find a public track or a flat, straight road.
- If you're running on a standard four-hundred-meter track, a mile is four laps.
- If you are on a road, you can map out your mile using a GPS watch or an app on your phone (I like Runkeeper). Jog out until you've hit a mile. Your test will be the run on the way back to where you started.
- Complete one warm-up mile, going slow and easy. If you're on a road, this can be your run to map out a mile. Stay relaxed. It's just to loosen up.
- Do the dynamic warm-up (page 25).
- Now line up. Aim to go as fast as you can—but remember, a mile is not a sprint. You want a steady, fast pace. If you are gasping for air in the first minute, you are going too fast (so slow down). The ideal effort

would be if you're breathing moderately hard and can speak in short sentences. Now go!

Now that you have your mile time, you can calculate your marathon race pace. (Your marathon race pace is the average time per mile you should run the marathon.) Jeff Galloway, Olympian and the grandfather of marathoning, calls this method the "Magic Mile."

Your Mile Time x 1.3 = Marathon Race Pace

Let's say your mile time was 9:13 (9 minutes and 13 seconds)

Let's convert 9:13 to seconds: (9 x 60) + 13 = 553 seconds

553 seconds x 1.3 = 718.9 seconds

718.9 seconds is your marathon race pace. Let's convert this into minutes and seconds:

718.9 seconds = 11 minutes and 58.9 seconds

So my marathon race pace is 11:59 (11 minutes and 59 seconds).

Using your one-mile time, you can calculate other paces that you'll need to know while training. The easiest and most foolproof way to find the pace you are supposed to run for any distance is to use the Jack Daniels' VDOT Running Calculator. This calculator is available via the VDOT Running Calculator app or on the Run S.M.A.R.T. Project website, https://runsmartpro ject.com/calculator/. There you can input your race distance and time. If you have a PR time from a 5K or longer race, you can take that number to determine various paces. If not, you can input your one-mile time. You can also input temperature (the hotter it is, the harder it is) and altitude (higher altitude makes it feel like you are breathing through a straw) if you want, which is why I like this running calculator more than others.

If you're using the Run S.M.A.R.T. Project website, after inputting your race distance and time into the calculator, you'll see three tabs appear. For right now, you'll want to focus on the second and third tabs, labeled "training" and "equivalent." Here's what you need to know.

I inputted that I ran a 5K in 24:35.

My training paces would be:

>   Easy and long:* 10:01–11:00 minutes per mile
>   Threshold:† 8:21 minutes per mile
>   Interval:‡ 7:42 minutes per mile
>   Repetition:§ 7:17 minutes per mile

My race paces, which, by the way, we might use in lieu of training paces on some speed days, would be:

>   Marathon: 8:56 minutes per mile
>   Half-marathon: 8:38 minutes per mile
>   10K: 8:13 minutes per mile
>   5K: 7:55 minutes per mile

The thing about training paces is that there is no hard-and-fast calculation that is agreed upon by mathematicians and runners alike. Jack Daniels is one of the most respected runners and coaches in the world and uses his formula to train both Olympians and pedestrian runners. Though Daniels is the gold standard, there are other pace calculators that work just as well to give you a range to aim for. There are apps like the VDOT Running Calculator, Track-Splits, and Pace Chase that will calculate run paces for free.

Time vs. Distance

If you're newer to running, many coaches recommend using a time to reach as a goal rather than distance. So instead of trying to reach six miles, your plan might call for a seventy-minute run. There are many reasons for trying

---

* Your long-run pace should be essentially the same as your easy-run pace; it could even be slightly slower.

† Threshold pace is the pace you'll want to use for the tempo test (page 85).

‡ Interval pace is the pace you'll want to use for the intervals test (page 79).

§ Repetition pace is the pace you'll want to use for the repeats test (page 81).

this method. First, too many runners focus on pace, no matter what anyone tells them. So if you are someone who gets hung up on time per mile, just paying attention to the number of minutes you run will take away the urge to look at your pace. In fact, the best way to get over your pace hang-up is to set a countdown timer and just run, without any data, until the buzzer sounds.

Physically, time is a better metric to consider if you're training at a slower pace. Once we get to in-season training, the long runs get longer. Many plans for intermediate and advanced runners call for twenty miles. That might not work with your pace. No one should be out on a road running for more than five hours trying to complete twenty miles. Even if it does take you that long on race day, that time spent running during training will take a toll on your body and could lead to sidelining injuries. The renowned coach Jack Daniels, a man who's coached for well over four decades and trained thirty-one NCAA DIII champions, made it a rule that nobody should be out on their long run for more than three hours.

The problem with that, of course, is that a runner using a 10:45 training pace, for example, will never make it to twenty miles in three hours. And yet the twenty-miler is something that many athletes feel is necessary to complete to feel mentally prepared for race day.

Many of us run twelve-minute miles for our easy pace, which would have us completing a twenty-miler in four hours. What would Daniels say about that? There are options here. First, you could split any runs more than three hours into two, running for three hours, stopping, waiting four to eight hours, then completing whatever you have left. You will still be running on tired legs, which is optimal for marathon prep, but they won't be so tired that you'll risk injury.

Some coaches are of the opinion that a four-hour twenty-miler isn't the end of the world. That's because the slower pace lessens the intensity and thus the risk. I say you have to make this decision for yourself. When you're deep into the run, around 2:30, begin scanning for pain or awkwardness (sloppy strides, shuffling instead of stepping), and stop when you feel it. No matter what, cap your workouts at four hours. You will still reap the aerobic benefits without placing too much strain on your muscles.

Mastering the Long Run

Running long can be intimidating for newer runners. Even seasoned pros can think about the eighteen-miler and get a little tense. Many veteran marathoners will admit to having a love-hate relationship with the all-powerful long run. These runs are everything—all-consuming, glorious, the highlight of your week, the thing that keeps you up at night. Embrace it all. These runs will, after all, make up the bulk of your weekly miles. When I started marathon training, I looked at the plan, saw the giant numbers representing long runs, and blindly followed directions without questioning why. I figured that the steady increase was preparing my body and mind for the eventual 26.2. But how did that happen?

Think about it: it's a miracle that we travel ten, twelve, eighteen miles on our own two feet. We know all the work is doing something, but what exactly is happening in our bodies? Knowing the long run's importance can only help us maximize our success.

I asked running coach Erica Coviello to explain the necessity of running long. Erica, as I mentioned earlier, is an exercise scientist and RRCA-certified coach. She specializes in beginning runners and midpackers who want to get stronger and faster. She is all about process and patience, and she expects her runners to put in the work while being smart (which means listening to her). "You have to teach your body to run for a long time. It doesn't just know how to do that right off the bat," she says. "Throughout the training, with each long run, you increase your aerobic capacity, stroke the volume of the heart, build muscle strength in every part of your legs, work ligaments, tendons, and synovial fluid. Your mind needs to be able to hack it too."

Ashlee Lawson Green, an RRCA-certified running coach and cofounder and CEO of RUNGRL, a platform for Black women that uses running as a vehicle to impact wellness, agrees: "It's not only getting time on the road and learning what to expect during the race, but mentally reaching past your limits and getting comfortable being in a new place, physically."

Both Erica and Ashlee have a knack for helping runners conquer those daunting long miles. Here are some of their tips and tricks to help you make it through.

Slow Down

The long run is an effort in and of itself—you shouldn't add the additional strain of running too fast. In fact, if you're doing your long runs at a pace that's not suitable for your aerobic capacity, the workout quickly turns into junk miles. Your body will rebel because it's overtaxed, and it won't be able to recover quickly enough for you to reap the benefits of your effort. With so much time and energy put into the long workouts, we must make them count.

Feeling like we need to go faster than we're physically capable of going can stem from a lot of things. You know, sometimes it feels really good to go fast. Sometimes we're just in a groove and we don't want to fight it. I completely understand this sentiment, but that pace that feels so right is actually too easy to be hard and too hard to be easy and so is not serving any actual purpose. I know that great, free feeling of zooming along with the wind in your hair, but if you want to feel that exuberance at the tail end of your run, hold yourself back just a bit.

The other issue, perhaps more common, is that many of us women are so task-oriented that it's only natural to want to go out and do the darn thing. We see a number on the training plan, and we go out and try to get through it as quickly as we possibly can. If this sounds like you, running by time rather than distance is a really good solution. You're allowed to give yourself space to train. Your long run should be just for you—and if you know you have to devote three hours of your weekend to it, you're more likely to take your time and enjoy it.

Finally, ego occasionally ruins our slow running. Again, we want to try to quiet our minds and get rid of that nagging internal voice that tells us we're running too slow. Sometimes the annoying voice creeps in when you glance down at your watch, and you want to pick up the pace. But hold on; you can reframe and reason with yourself. Remind yourself that your slow miles actually lead to faster times when it counts. Let go of the judgment of what is fast and what is slow. Say, "I'm running this pace now so I can run faster on race day." Be kind and gentle to your body.

Run with Friends

Coach Erica says that finding a group of runners to run long with provides the ultimate accountability. Whether that's joining a running club or finding a few pals who want to run for more than two hours, it helps to run with people of a similar pace who can slow down if the group starts getting too out of breath.

Virtual Pacer

Joining a running club might not be an option for everyone. Maybe you live in a place without a group. Or, like me, you can't fathom talking to people for that long. Coach Ashlee says that for her, running in a group setting actually makes her too fast. So if you need some accountability but not the people, a virtual pacer really helps. Most of the apps that offer this allow you to set the intended distance and the amount of time it should take you, and then they do the rest of the work to keep you in check. I really like Pace To Race and Pace Control.

Sound Changes

Music is an excellent distraction on long runs, but sometimes our music choices prime our bodies to go out way too fast. Pump-up music can increase heat rate and boost neurotransmitters, so that we feel like superheroes. If your playlist is too many beats per minute, it can mess up your breathing and turn-over. Save those songs for when you're working on speed (such as for tempo runs). For the long runs, try no music (safer) or podcasts (educational!), or curate a list of slower tunes.

Prehydrate

You can't expect to make it through a long run without proper hydration. And no, carrying a water bottle on your run will not cut it. For the two days prior to the long run, track your water intake. Count the number of ounces you drink. Eight eight-ounce glasses are recommended. Try to reach that minimum.

Have a Specific Plan

When thinking about your long run, some of the planning should be simple. First and foremost, you can't just wing it. Determine where you will run. Then think about what time of day you want to run. That's the most basic planning you can do.

If there's a specific marathon you'd like to run, it's smart to try to replicate some of what you'll face on race day. If you haven't even thought about a race yet, no sweat. Bookmark this page and come back once you have a race in mind.

When I say replicate the course, I mean you want to pay attention to the miles or areas that might give you problems. If you live close to the race-course, that's ideal. You can train on different segments each week.

If you're planning to travel to your race, as many runners do, you can check out course maps and incorporate hills, turns, flats, and water stops. This is a good idea for every runner, and it can get more granular the more advanced you are.

Say you're running the Marine Corps Marathon (MCM). Hopefully you chose this race because your running style matches the style of this course. For now, let's just say you chose very wisely because you needed a flatish course and the elevation map for MCM was perfect-o for you.

You can tell that it's a pretty flat course because the elevation range shown on the map is 0–230 feet, which is basically nothing—not a super hilly course. But there are a few rollers in there, notably at the beginning, at about mile eight, and then a small incline near the finish, which will feel like a monster just because it is at the end. So for some of your training runs, you might start with a gradual climb up and a nice downhill, then find another climb about a quarter of the way in, and then end with a big uphill.

If you want to get very down to details, figuring out the grades of hills on the course and matching them with your nearby hills can certainly build preparedness and confidence. To do this, turn to the Hill Test section on page 82.

Next you should map out water stations along the course if you're planning to use them as your main source of hydration. If you're running by distance, take in water when you plan to take it in during the race. The same goes for fuel.

Turns are also something to think about. MCM has a fair number of twists, a sharp U-turn at the literal halfway point, and curves at the end. You might not be able to replicate the course turn by turn, but you can incorporate a few changes of direction, not only to condition your leg and abdominal muscles but also to use the turns to your advantage mentally—instead of, for example, letting a midpoint turnaround get you too excited (like "Woo-hoo! I'm halfway there!" only to realize that the second half of the race is way harder and takes you to a lonely highway before spitting you back out into the middle of the city) or too defeated (like "This is halfway? I have so much to go!"). Finding a perfect balance between these two mind-sets is crucial. In your head, think of each turn as an exciting, new mini section of the course, and use this strategy as you train.

Test Your Fuel

Remember, taking in calories while you're running is a must if you're running for more than ninety minutes. Fueling options are based on the individual's taste and gastrointestinal tolerance. Meaning: you don't want to try something new on race day and have it backfire. If you have never eaten while running before, don't fear, you don't have to pack a calzone to eat at mile six. Exercise scientists and nutritionists have invented calorie-rich gels and gummies enriched with vitamins, and sometimes caffeine, that come in a variety of flavors. They come in packets small enough to tuck inside pockets. You have months to test different gels, drinks, gummies, and jelly beans. You can experiment with supplements that contain caffeine or drinks that replenish your electrolytes. Toss what doesn't work and keep what makes you feel good. Ideally, you will consume the fuel at similar times during every long run and replicate this timing on race day.

For example, one runner might take in calories near water stops at the following times: 0:15, 0:45, 1:30, 2:15, 3:00, 3:45, 4:30, and so on until they cross the finish line. In this fueling scenario, you'll notice that you take in fuel fifteen minutes into the race, you take in fuel again after another thirty minutes, and then you take in fuel every forty-five minutes after that. This is a good practice for people with nervous stomachs, because you get calories in early, then let that first dose settle, then resume in a normal pattern. This is to say that you should test out different fueling strategies in practice to see what works for you. You might find that your stomach cannot handle the fuel so often, so you might increase the amount of time between snacks. You might also want to try eating more often as time passes. I know that when things get hairy three hours and forty-five minutes in, eating calories and caffeine makes me feel like a superwoman for, well, like, maybe thirty seconds. No matter what your on-the-run eating habits look like, try to consume something at least every forty-five minutes.

Dress the Part

Many runners skip this suggestion, but it's imperative that you test out what you're going to wear on race day! Seriously. Nobody wants to be surprised by an unsupportive sports bra or shorts that chafe.

There are a great number of accessories on the market for us. Some are really useful—fuel belts, for example, are essential to most marathoners. They fit around your waist and hold your choice of snack, sometimes a phone, Band-Aids, and anything you might need that can fit in a small pocket. Some people prefer vests that do the same thing. Still others like hydration backpacks that have a bladder in the pack and a straw, so that your water is with you at all times. No matter what you prefer, test it on a training run.

Listen to Your Body (and Not Always Your Brain)

Running long is tough. It's going to hurt. Every coach I talked to expressed this same sentiment: you cannot escape the pain of marathon training. So it's essential, even on your shorter long runs, for you to know how to tell the difference between your brain telling you to stop and physical fatigue. In the former scenario, you have to train the mind to shut up and let you keep rolling. In the latter, though, you actually should stop, because grinding it out could lead to injury—or a week afterward that is pointless because your body cannot recover quickly enough. When you're in mile seven and you feel like your feet are encased in concrete, some runners might say, "That's it," and call it quits even though there is nothing physically wrong. Others might plow through, only to suffer the consequences afterward. So how do you know?

"Both are hurdles that suck to get over, but both are conquerable," Coach Erica says. "You're going to be tired, but you can be tired and still move efficiently. Moderately tired muscles will recover with rest. But lousy form or pain from an injury is more problematic. Improper form leads to injuries, and injuries only get worse when you keep running on them."

The key to determining which you're dealing with is honesty. Scan your body. Is there actual pain? If so, stop. If you think it's a mental block, pause for a moment. Admire your surroundings and think about all the miles you've accomplished so far. Take some deep breaths. Now here's the key: start running again at a slower pace than you were going before. Try a run-walk for ten minutes, alternating thirty seconds of walking with thirty seconds of running. But if you are straining to breathe or you notice your form is wobbly, then you might consider taking a longer rest—like a minute.

No matter what, if you need to stop short on your long run day, it's OK. But don't reschedule those miles on a rest day. Remind yourself that your body needed a break, and you'll come back stronger on the next scheduled long run.

Recover Right Afterward

Yes, long-run days should include naps. If you don't have time to rest and recover, then you're not properly training. Your postrun routine should include some other acts of self-care. A long shower, a body scan, nursing any battle wounds, icing troublesome areas, keeping your lower extremities elevated, and eating delicious recovery-day meals should all be on your long-run-day checklist. Go to bed early and thank your body for all the hard work it accomplished.

Keep Recovering

Coach Erica believes programming a rest day after a long run is beneficial for recovery. On this delightful day after the long run, you might find yourself even more exhausted than you were the day of the run. It's normal. But don't let that exhaustion keep you in bed all day. Instead, live by the three w's on these days: walk (slowly for twenty minutes), water (drink it!), and wait (to run again). If you are feeling tight, stretching can help. Don't push it too hard, though. An hour of vinyasa yoga is not resting. Focus on simple movements: While standing, lift your arms overhead with your fingers reaching toward the sky, and breathe. Fold over and touch your toes. Roll your neck, shoulders, wrists, and ankles. Do what feels good to your body.

Leveling Up

By now, I'm certain you're sick of hearing the old "slow down" mantra—especially if you're a marathoner with a strong base and a few races under your belt. When you get to the in-season training plans, advanced runners will see distance runs punctuated with "race pace" miles. That means you will run some miles at the same time you're planning to run your goal race. I'll explain more about this once you're through the base training plan.

Coach Erica talks about how individual this process can be for each athlete and each situation. In one recent case, she altered a plan slightly based on knowledge, data, and instinct.

"When my client and I first talked about her goals, she wanted to get to the finish line uninjured," Coach Erica recalls. "She is an avid marathoner, so we knew that a cherry on top would be making it to the finish a smidge faster than her PR. We didn't actually set a goal time, because she was just finishing up some PT for an injury and didn't want to jump into much intensity. By the time she made it to a long run that required sixteen miles, she'd been given the all-clear by her doc. I was watching closely too, and I saw she was totally rocking every single run. I decided that it was time to add some intensity and programmed five race-pace miles into the sixteen-miler, which is rare. I usually plug them in during the eighteen-miler."

Erica's intimate knowledge of her athlete's body, plan, and progress allowed her to make a call that helped not just physically but mentally. "It showed me that she was capable of exactly what I think she's capable of [i.e., a massive PR]. More importantly, it gave her the confidence to set a time goal and continue moving forward with a plan to chase it down. She ended up running a twenty-four-minute PR."

But adding race-pace miles at any time during the long run is not something she recommends for a beginner or intermediate athlete, unless you have a coach monitoring you. "For runners aiming for anything longer than a 3:45 time goal," she says, "it isn't worth the risk. I usually program some marathon-pace (or faster) miles during midweek runs."

Finally, Trust Yourself

Trust the process and the professionals, but more important, trust yourself. For the most part, as long as you're injury free, your body can handle the long run and the build. It's your brain that you need to train. Accept that it's hard, and appreciate yourself for doing hard things.

Quick Tips to Get You Through When You Just Can't Even

Pick a new place to run.

Run your usual route backward.

Join a local running club.

Buy some new clothes or gear to motivate you!

Hop on a trail.

Take photos along the way.

Think about it in chunks, e.g., just five miles four times!

Run the mile you're in.

Be like Kipchoge and smile!*

---

* Do you know Eliud Kipchoge? He's a professional marathoner and the first runner who ran a sub-two-hour marathon, a barrier that people once thought impossible to break. Anyway, that's all well and good, but the best part about him is the fact that he smiles while he runs. He runs for the pure joy of it. His outlook is contagious.

A Few Warnings

Listen, if you're new to running several miles at a time, I'm going to tell you that there are some horror stories to be aware of. Well, *horror stories* might be a little bit strong, but there are some not-so-pleasant things that can happen to your body when out for a run. So let's get those out of the way now.

My friend Erin, who is much speedier than I will ever be, once told me about a wonderful run that turned into her worst nightmare. She'd recently switched to a diet with more fiber—she felt healthier and filled with more energy, but her system was still adjusting to the change. She went out for a long training run in her neighborhood, which is a sunlit, utopian farming community with rolling country roads that go on forever. She felt great at the outset of the run, which was scheduled to be a fifteen-miler. It was a hot day and she was wearing just a sports bra and tiny running shorts. Somewhere around mile seven, she felt a rumbling in her stomach that quickly turned into a cramp. She figured that it would go away, because you can often keep running, pass gas, and continue onward. But soon she felt a terrible weight pressing down on her bowels. She leaped off the road into a cornfield and struggled to get her shorts down fast enough. In her telling, it was a literal sh*tstorm. So yes, the rumors are true, poop happens. At some point during your training, even if you're eating perfectly, you will likely feel intestinal distress. That urgent poop is likely a result of your colon being stimulated by the up-and-down movement of running. Running also takes blood to the hardest-working parts of your body first, before sending it to the GI tract. This can cause that sudden need to poop, as well as stomach cramps, pain, and diarrhea. What joy.

Erin is a trooper. She thought fast and removed one of the pads in her sports bra to use as toilet paper. She did not feel great. Wisely, she decided to turn back toward home and called her partner to pick her up from her walk of shame.

The key here, and with all situations in your long run, is to plan. Test out the fuel you plan to use. Try out the meals you want to eat the night and morning before. If you learn that you're prone to this type of thing, plan a route with available bathrooms. Or plan to bring toilet paper. Plan not to go to the bathroom in your neighbor's yard.

What else? Peeing is common, especially in women who've given birth and are working toward strengthening their pelvic floor. If this is you, see page 148 in chapter nine, because there are remedies!

Anyway, there's other gnarly stuff to look out for. Chafing happens. Your inner thighs might get raw. There are products like Body Glide and Vaseline—basically lube for running—that you can use on any of the sensitive areas that rub when you run.

Maybe more intimidating than anything is the fear of the unknown. Every long run is different and presents its own challenges, but be prepared to surprise yourself. Many people who do multiple marathons fall in love with the process and cherish the hours they spend grinding out the long run. This is where champions are born.

MORE TESTS!

If you take a look at your base training schedule, you'll see a few "test" days (intervals test, repeats test, hill test, tempo test, VO2 max test). I want to assure you that none of these workouts will be, in my opinion, half as bad as the Magic Mile test. Actually, I think you will be pleasantly surprised. Base training can get a little boring with all that building and restraint in terms of pace and mileage. But the tests can be fun and give you insights into your running style. Plus, identifying your strengths and strengthening your weaknesses can be the key to unlocking your running potential. Many women who run start not with the goal of getting quicker but instead to find peace, lose weight, develop a hobby, recover from addiction, make themselves healthier, or boost their self-esteem. But at a certain point, many of us want to up the ante. We don't just want to finish a marathon; we want to set a new personal best.

Here's the thing: I know a lot of women who go out and run race after race, only to come up short of their goals. They may shave off a minute here and there, but it's not a massive improvement. Even if time is just an external goal, the outcome could play a part in how you feel about your intrinsic goal, and that's totally natural and valid. With subpar results, you might feel like you're stuck in a rut. Runners who go through the motions of training time and time again and then run a race at the same level they've been running since they were beginners might start to wonder what they're doing wrong.

While I can't see into your training life, I can address some of the most common issues experienced coaches see. A huge portion of marathoners simply don't have enough variation in their training. For example, my pal Julie, also known as the Marathon Goddess, is a master's athlete who started her running journey when she was thirty-seven years old. Once she ran her first marathon, she fell in love with the distance and then spent three years with finishing times anywhere between 4:15 and 5:30. That was good enough for her. She had traded most of her self-destructive vices for a pair of running shoes. But as she started hanging out with runners more frequently, she kept hearing about this magical pilgrimage to Boston. What is Boston? Why do you have to qualify? What time do I need to run to get in? The allure of the Boston Marathon gets implanted in so many runners' minds. It's an incredible goal, a gateway into amateur elitism. But getting in shape to run a Boston qualifying time is, well, really freaking hard. Julie didn't really adjust anything in her training except for mileage volume. She truly believed that if she just ran more, she could get there. Hundreds of miles and eleven marathons later, she was at a loss. She consulted a coach (finally).

He looked at her training logs and joined her for a ten-miler. He could see two problems immediately:

1. There was absolutely no speed work in her plans.
2. She was running her long runs too fast, going at about a nine-minute pace when that was too far above her aerobic threshold.

In fact, she ran every mile around this pace—a pace that she said felt "good." She hated (still hates, actually) track workouts. Track workouts, for all my speed-work virgins out there, are faster-paced running routines. Usually they include short bursts of medium-hard to hard runs, followed by a limited rest period where you either walk or do a slow recovery jog. We call them track workouts because they're usually performed on a track, but they can be done on a road. Anyway, my friend avoided the old oval (cool slang for *track*) at all costs. She'd never tried exercises to push her speed endurance (such as tempo runs, which I'll explain soon), and when she slowed her long-run pace down to the suggested 11:30, she said she basically wanted to die. Nevertheless, she listened to her coach—she slowed down her long-run pace and added weekly sessions at the track. And guess what? She qualified for Boston.

How? Well, the combination of running to improve her aerobic base plus recruiting her fast-twitch muscles and anaerobic capabilities through exercises such as intervals, repeats, hills, and tempo runs was key to making her a better marathon runner. Those changes, the alternating slower and faster paces, paid off.

If you take one thing away from this, just remember that you cannot do the same thing every single day and expect to improve. And you certainly cannot do solely what makes you feel good. A little bit of discomfort mixed with a dash of something new and weird will help you grow. Now it's time to find out what your body is capable of and how we can fine-tune your training so that it addresses your deficits!

As you go through these tests, I want you to pay attention to the following elements and be ready to record them:

> **Rate of perceived exertion (RPE)** is a numeric value you assign to how hard you feel you're working. Starting at zero (I'm sitting on my couch) and capping off at ten (everything hurts and I'm dying), you use this number to assess how hard you're working. In an ideal world, your easy days would feel like a three and your harder days would be a seven or eight. As you go through the tests, at the hardest moment, try to rate how you're feeling. Two things here: If you are truly feeling like you're running a ten, back off a bit. Almost nothing should feel like a ten. But hey, don't say you're redlining at ten every time if you are not. RPE is a great way to assess your level of fitness, but it only works if you are honest with yourself. So rate yourself accurately. As you go, you can

compare each workout with what your hardest effort has been to date.

Breath. Can you do these workouts while maintaining a controlled breath pattern? Are you literally gasping for air at any point? These tests will likely leave you out of breath at some point. Pay attention to how hard it is for you to recover a steady breath pattern.

Average heart rate is a good indicator of how hard you're working. In addition to what your heart rate registers at the end of your workout, pay attention to both its peak and how long it takes you to recover.

Feelings will contribute to performance. Bring an emotional awareness to your run. Check in at the beginning, middle, and end of each test. Don't worry if you forget how you were feeling in the middle—you might just be fatigued enough to not feel any type of way. I think I would call that "immersed" or "determined" or perhaps just plain old "exhausted." In any case, write down two to three words that describe how you felt while completing the exercise or how you feel about the exercise overall. You might feel "anxious" or "strong" and "mad as heck" that you have to run ten hills.

Once you've made it through each of the tests below, do what you need to do to recover properly. That means light stretching, refueling and replenishing, and rehydrating. The next morning, run some diagnostics on your body.

A read of your resting **heart rate** in the morning is a good indicator of how much strain your body endured. If it's much higher than normal, the workout may have left you overexerted.

Rate **how you feel physically** on a scale from zero (I feel like an unstoppable she-wolf) to ten (I feel like a she-wolf ripped my legs off). **Fatigue** can be measured in the same way, though you should wait until about 2:00 p.m. to see if you're drained or feeling pretty OK overall. You will have either a rest day or a slow-run day after the test. Measuring your RPE on an easy run is a great litmus test for just how much the previous day's test affected you.

Track Workouts (aka Speed Work)

Intervals Test

Interval workout 8 x 800

Intervals are short and intense runs followed by a period of cardiovascular rest. In this workout, you'll be running a half mile (eight hundred meters) eight times with a ninety-second jog in between. These ninety-second jogs are active recovery, which means that you can catch your breath and lower your heart rate while still moving and keeping your blood pumping. Active recovery really helps with endurance.

If you have access to a public track, head over there (check your local middle and high schools). An eight hundred is two laps around, assuming the oval near you is a standard four-hundred-meter outdoor track. If you don't have a track, you simply need a flat stretch of road and maybe a piece of chalk. If you don't have chalk, a rock will do! Don't overthink it. Pick a starting point and measure a quarter of a mile out. Mark it so you have something visual to refer to that isn't your watch. That will be your turnaround point.

Devote about five minutes to the classic dynamic warm-up. Next complete a mile-long warm-up at a very easy pace. Now your body is ready.

Run the first eight hundred at a quick pace, but it must be a pace you can sustain until the end of the workout. Keep your eyes fixed slightly ahead of you and up. Don't look at the ground, to the side, or behind you. The eyeline is important in speed work to maintain forward progression and focus. Even though you're going to run faster than your normal easy days, your hands should remain relaxed, like you're holding baby birds. We don't want to change your form too much, but do think of the knee drive as your propelling force. Speed requires more of a forefoot strike (landing more on the ball or middle portion of your foot) as opposed to a heel strike (landing on your heels). This isn't a short sprint, so it shouldn't look much different from your easy-run form, but thinking about it in terms of forward momentum will help you push a little faster. Keep your neck and shoulders relaxed, and engage your arm swing. Often, if you hold your arms close to your body (keep your elbows in, or else you risk running like a Muppet!), your legs will follow in the same line, which creates a more efficient stride.

If you're using a pace calculator, you should aim to run at your interval pace. If you don't know your interval pace, each interval should feel challenging but not like you're gasping for air. You should be breathing heavily and using the 2:1 breath pattern (see page 103). The effort should be manageable, meaning—and I cannot say this enough—don't go out too fast. You'll want to time each interval as well as your rest time. That ninety-second recovery is actually the interval that's important here. You won't fully recover—and you don't want to—but it will give you a chance to catch your breath.

We do intervals for speed endurance. They stress your VO2 max (more on this soon). By pushing your body to its limit, then backing off, then doing it again, you increase both aerobic and anaerobic capacity simultaneously. The intervals also bring your fast-twitch muscles to the party. Intervals are exhausting, exhilarating, and one of the most effective ways to improve your speed and confidence.

If this is your strength: You are speedy and this kind of workout probably feels fun. Maybe it feels like you are flying. You can add to the challenge and work on form, turnover, strength, and speed by incorporating advanced interval workouts, which you'll soon read about, during your in-season training. If this is your strength but you learn or know that turns are your weakness, then make the following adjustments: If you are using a track, consider moving off the track to a stretch of road to better simulate what you'll be running on race day and to get the feel of a very sharp turn at the halfway point.

If this is your weakness: Intervals might be one of the most challenging exercises runners put themselves through. Identify what is hard about it. If you're having trouble pushing yourself but not feeling fatigued at the end, then you could find a fast friend to help pace you. If you're feeling like you're about to collapse, then you likely went out too hard, and you can plan to pace yourself better next time. Guess what? I bet 90 percent of people who think intervals are impossible are simply running too hard off the bat. I encourage you to utilize a pace calculator and use your Magic Mile time or time from your last race (within the past three months) to get an idea of the kind of pace at which you need to be running your intervals. This could change your life.

No matter what the perceived difficulty is, you will likely see results fast if you incorporate interval training into your routine.

Repeats Test

Repeats workout 6 x 400

Repeats are short and intense runs with a period of cardiovascular rest that is typically longer than the rest period in an interval workout. Four hundreds are commonly called quarters because four hundred meters is a quarter of a mile. In this workout, you will be running six four hundreds with a four-hundred-meter active recovery in between each repeat. Go to your track or the stretch of road where you marked the quarter mile for the interval test. You can use the same tips from running intervals. They all apply.

Complete the dynamic warm-up, followed by a one-mile warm-up run. You will be running four hundred meters six times. Run each of the four hundreds at your repetition (repeats) pace, or roughly the same pace at which you ran your intervals. After you run each four hundred, you can do a light jog for two hundred meters and then walk the remaining two hundred meters back to the start line. Don't worry about timing yourself during this rest period. In doing so, your heart rate should drop to about sixty percent of its max.

Repeats are very similar to intervals with the exception of the rest period. Giving yourself more recovery allows you to run the following repeat as hard as or harder than you ran the previous one. Maintaining your initial effort for every repetition is a great way to train step cadence and improve leg turnover speed. Short-burst repetitions like these four hundreds enhance pure speed more than speed endurance but contribute to the improvement of both. You might not think track speed is important when running 26.2, but shaving a few seconds off each mile will take minutes off your time. Remember, all those seconds add up!

If this is your strength: Then you are a beast. You are a track star in the making. You will probably find your stride on courses with long straights, especially if those straights happen toward the end of the race. Your finishing kick will be legendary, meaning you will be able to accelerate at the end of the race and zoom at superspeed to the finish line. However, a lot of people who run speedy short distances go too fast on easy days and long runs just because they can.

If this is your weakness: Mentally, repetitions are tough. You recover enough that your thinking mind will want to be done. Even your physical body nears the point of being relaxed and feels like "Cool, great job today, let's leave the track." But then you put your toes to the line again, and your mind and body feel tormented, like you are just messing with them and their flow! If your legs are getting tired before your breath is, that means you're doing it right. Push through that soreness! But if you're getting out of breath and unable to sustain the same pace on reps two and three, then you likely need to set a slower pace for each of your four hundreds—and that's fine. It will still get you results. Anyway, if you master these grueling repeats, your mind will be able to handle the emotional roller coaster that is a marathon. And you *will* get faster. It does not matter if you were always last in the fifty-yard dash in grade school. Now is your chance at redemption. Repeats are designed to make you speedy beyond your wildest dreams.

Hill Test

First things first. How do you calculate the grade of a hill? First you'll need a run tracker or GPS watch to measure elevation and distance. The grade is the vertical gain divided by the distance of the hill you're covering. Go out to a hill. Track both distance and elevation gain in feet. Grab a calculator.

> Let's say you gained 200 feet and you did this over 0.5 miles.
> First convert the mileage to feet. There are 5,280 feet in a mile.
> 0.5 x 5,280 = 2,640 feet
> Then divide the amount of gain (200 feet) by that distance:
> 200 feet of gain / 2,640 feet = about 0.076
> That's a hill with a 7.6 percent grade. The higher the grade, the
> steeper the hill.

If you live in Kansas and there is nothing near you that even vaguely resembles an ascent, you have a few options: treadmill (safest), parking garage (basically the same thing as the road but runs the risk of getting you hit by a car), and stairs or bleachers (fun but very difficult).

There are a few key elements in hill-running form.

1. Your body should hinge forward slightly at the hips.
2. Run close to the balls of your feet. This could be your forefoot or literally your toes. Really, you will be able to feel it out. Just don't stomp up to the top on your heels. That's akin to driving uphill with the emergency brake on.
3. Bring your knees up in a more exaggerated way than if you were running on flat land. Engage your glutes by squeezing your cheeks. Not only will this wake them up and ensure you aren't overstressing your hamstrings and quads, but it will strengthen this muscle group in a similar way to air squats. Cool, right? But don't stop continuing to practice your squats!
4. Your arms' swing should mimic your legs'. Pump them to produce power from your biceps.
5. Relax your shoulders! Seriously, drop them down from your ears. Shake them out. They want to creep up, but don't let them. That uses too much energy.
6. Keep your neck long, the crown of your head pointed toward the top of the incline, and your eyes gazing toward the ground two to three steps ahead. Some prefer to look at the top of the hill, but this can be defeating. You can try both options and see what works best for you.

OK, now that you know the form and have your hill picked out, you're ready to go.

Long Hill Repeats 6 x 2 minutes

In this workout, you will be running uphill for two minutes, then downhill for two minutes, six times. Find a stretch of road—or grass or trail—on a hill with a 4 percent grade. If you have a very long hill available, or a series of hills, that will help.

Warm up by doing a slow mile at your easiest pace on flat land to get your blood pumping, and then complete the dynamic warm-up.

Next, set your watch to stopwatch mode. For the next two minutes, run up the hill at your 10K pace. It should be slower than your 5K pace but feel similar in effort. When you're done running uphill for two minutes, turn around and run downhill. You should also give yourself about two minutes to reach the bottom of the hill. The downhill portion should be relatively easy. Push on the uphill, float on the down. Back at the starting point, walk for ninety seconds. Repeat five more times.

If you add one hard effort into your training plan, make it be hills. Hills are an amazing tool because they offer both variety and intensity. Every hill is different. Every hill is hard. Get over it. (Dad joke!) Really, though, every single hill is not only surmountable but improves your power, endurance, anaerobic capacity, speed, and overall strength. Training on hills is the only workout that uses slow-, intermediate-, and fast-twitch muscles. When you use the correct form, you run close to the balls of your feet, which makes your calves turn into machines. Your knees pump higher, so your stride gets more powerful and the major muscles in your core engage. Squeeze those cheeks and hello, booty gains. All this translates to making you a faster, more efficient, and more well-rounded runner.

If this is your strength: You're like me! I love hills. Maybe you have a naturally strong trunk and butt. You might embrace the challenge of scrambling up steep grades. Or maybe you love the visual satisfaction of seeing just how high you climbed. Whatever it is, a racecourse with rolling hills might be an excellent choice for you. Just because you lose momentum going up doesn't mean you can't make up for any lost time by flying back down. Of course, going downhill can be just as tiring as the ascent, so if you're looking to amp up your hill game, doing short hill repeats with effort on both the climb and the descent will get your legs in hill-crushing shape.

If this is your weakness: Welp, that's not that uncommon. Hills can get in your head. And they can also get to your breath. There are a lot of misconceptions about how to conquer low- and midgrade hills that often lead to unnecessary fatigue. First, maintain a pace that allows you to keep a steady breath. If you're pushing the hills, as in a workout, breathe in for two steps and then out for one. If you encounter a hill on a long run or easy workout, keep the pace to where you can still talk. If you have to walk up in order for that to happen, that's all right. Second, a lot of our hatred of hills comes from our own darn heads. We see them coming and we get scared or annoyed or angry. Reframe that. Look at a hill as a challenge that will only prove your amazing strength. Conquer it, and if you're given a downhill, let loose and let gravity carry you to the bottom. The only way hills get easier is if you run them frequently. If you add them into your easy-run routes and make them your go-to for hard days, you will learn to love them.

Tempo Test

10-minute tempo

Get ready to run at a very uncomfortable pace for ten minutes, because that's what this test entails. Your tempo runs are completed at what is called lactate threshold. Research has shown that the lactate threshold occurs at 80 to 90 percent of your maximum heart rate in trained athletes and 60 percent in beginners.

If you're not an exercise scientist or glued to your heart rate monitor, let's just say that your rate of perceived exertion (RPE) should be around a six or seven—meaning it should feel tough but not impossible.

Don't just go from zero to one hundred. You want to prime your body for the effort. First get your heart rate going with ten jumping jacks and your dynamic warm-up. Then run easy for ten minutes. Amp it up to tempo pace, which some pace calculators refer to as threshold pace, and hold for ten minutes. At the end of your hard-effort time, shift down to an easy jog for the last ten minutes.

Listen, if you get to five minutes and crash, that's OK. Take a walk break for two minutes, then run at an easy pace for two minutes, then rev your engine up to tempo (but a bit slower than before) for another five minutes.

If you're advanced and tempo runs have been in your wheelhouse for a few training cycles, do a three-mile tempo for this test. If that seems easy, this is clearly your strength.

Tempo runs will help you master speed endurance, with the emphasis on endurance. Science will tell you that this workout is intended to push your lactate threshold to the limit, so that your blood must clear lactate at a faster rate than it's used to. Eventually these runs will make you faster and give you the superpower of sustaining a faster pace for longer.

If this is your strength: You love to feel the burn! You're likely a masochist. Kidding! I'm so proud of you for embracing this type of workout. Because there is no external obstacle or visual finish line and you have to maintain a pace that is painful for a longish period of time, this takes incredible mental stamina. The good news is that you are already comfortable with being uncomfortable, which is the name of the game in marathoning. So where do you go from here? Increasing your hard-effort time is a start. Intermediate runners should start increasing the tempo time by minute-long increments. If you get stuck at a certain point (like, say, ten minutes was easy but twelve minutes is really tough), then drop down at that breaking point to a walk or a jog. Recover. Then try to go for five minutes more at tempo pace. If you're an advanced runner, adding a series of ten-minute tempo-pace bursts to the middle miles of your long run will challenge you and might make your goal pace feel easy-breezy.

If this is your weakness: It takes both supreme physical fitness and mega mental fortitude to run at the lactate threshold pace. If this feels impossible, that's totally normal. When you see advanced runners doing tempo workouts, they will likely be doing them for thirty to forty minutes at a time. But you don't have to go out and run at that hard pace for thirty minutes if you've never done this before. That's why the test is short and sweet. Just like when you first began running, start small and work up to it. Try to sustain your tempo pace for as long as you can, then ask yourself to give fifteen seconds more. The following week, add a minute to the number you achieved the week before. Build like this for a few weeks and you'll surprise yourself. The strangest thing about tempo runs, which I experience and which I've heard from many runners, is that you can sustain a slightly faster pace in 5K races without stopping, but when you are alone, without someone to pass or other people's eyes on you, it's really tough to sustain that hard of a pace. Doing tempo runs with friends will help. It might still suck, but you will see massive gains while building a crazy amount of grit.

VO2 Max Test

Finally, let's talk about the main measurement of running performance. Generally, physiologists would turn to VO2 max, which is your body's ability to consume oxygen. The more oxygen your body takes in while at its maximum capacity to perform, the better.

A lot of things contribute to this number. The number of red blood cells you have and the amount of blood your heart can pump per minute when running will affect a VO2 reading. So how do you know your number?

You could go to a controlled lab setting and get hooked up to a bunch of tubes and wires. In the lab, the white coats can measure ventilation, oxygen, and carbon dioxide concentration of both inhaled and exhaled air. It might sound extreme, but that's truly the only way to get an accurate read.

I'm guessing most of you don't have a team of physiologists and sports doctors around, so testing VO2 accurately will be a struggle. But we can get a baseline snapshot with an at-home test. If anything, these tests are really great to see where your aerobic capacity is and provide a benchmark to see how you're progressing while training. Also, they're wicked fun.

Balke Test

Go to your track or a flat road where you'll be able to track the distance you covered. Set a stopwatch for fifteen minutes. Run as hard as you can for the fifteen-minute duration. Measure the distance covered in meters and throw it into this equation:

$$VO2 = 0.172 \times (meters/15 - 133) + 33.3$$

So if I wanted to put myself through this test, I might run 3,200 meters in fifteen minutes, on a good day. Here is what the calculation would look like:

$$VO2 = 0.172 \times (3,200/15 - 133) + 33.3$$
$$VO2 = 0.172 \times (80.3) + 33.3$$

$$VO2 = 13.81 + 33.3$$
$$VO2 = 47.1$$

Here is the chart that would tell me where my score falls:

Maximal Oxygen Uptake Norms for Women

	Age (years)					
rating	18–25	26–35	36–45	46–55	56–65	65+
excellent	> 56	> 52	> 45	> 40	> 37	> 32
good	47–56	45–52	38–45	34–40	32–37	28–32
above average	42–46	39–44	34–37	31–33	28–31	25–27
average	38–41	35–38	31–33	28–30	25–27	22–24
below average	33–37	31–34	27–30	25–27	22–24	19–21
poor	28–32	26–30	22–26	20–24	18–21	17–18
very poor	<28	<26	<22	<20	<18	<17

Again, this won't give you an exact read, but it will give you a decent idea of where you are. Despite the numbers, you can see that this test would vary based on conditions and your motivation on that day.

But I know what you're thinking now: How do I improve that number? Intervals are really effective—but any of the anaerobic workouts (think: hills, tempo runs, repeats) you put yourself through will help in different ways.

Now you have the knowledge of what your body prefers. Working on the stuff that isn't quite your jam will only make you a stronger, more well-rounded runner. But keep in mind that there is a recipe for success in your training plans. You can't just throw in workouts willy-nilly. The important thing is to build your strength and mileage in a smart way. Going too far or too fast will lead to injury. What I mean to say is that when these faster workouts are also longer, it's very hard on your muscles and joints. So to be safe, follow the training plans.

Now that we've covered the basics of base training, I want to introduce you to some things that will bolster your running experience. We've got a lot of work to do, and your body and mind need to be ready.

CHAPTER 7

TRAIN YOUR BRAIN

The key to performance in any athletic pursuit is the mind-body connection. Many runners think they can skip this part. They might think they are already mentally strong and that their brains don't suffer from the pitfalls of their more neurotic friends. The truth is, everyone can benefit from working on the mental aspect of marathoning.

The main goal of this chapter is to help you build a mental awareness of your physical body. The more tuned in we are to the sensations in our body, the more equipped we are to overcome the fatigue and pain we will inevitably feel during marathon training. And by opening up the lines of communication between our mental and physical selves, we will be able to quiet our minds so that our bodies can function to their maximum ability.

So let's wake up our awareness and start to notice our physical beings. Yeah, OK, it sounds a little new age—but when you're hobbling down the road at mile twenty-four with a cramp in your calf that just won't ease up, you will be grateful that you have these tips stored in your brain.

TAKE INVENTORY

In the exercises below, I'm going to show you how to take a body inventory. It's very simple. You just need five to ten minutes to rest on your back and think about each body part and how it feels. While it sounds pretty elementary, many people are surprised by the information a simple body scan delivers. You might be ignoring a tight hamstring or powering through a slight ache in your low back. Maybe your mouth feels dry. Maybe you're dehydrated and didn't even notice. These little ailments might seem like nothing, but with the load you put on your body during training, they might get worse. Or with proper prehab and strength work, they might get better. After noticing these ailments, you can enact solutions. Little tensions, like pain from hunched shoulders, can be remedied with a bit of attention and a few deep breaths. But for right now, just observe. Focus on noticing how every part of your body feels.

Exercise 1

Lie down on your back and make yourself as comfortable as possible. Starting with your head and face, focus on each body part one at a time. If you are on a muscle or muscle group, contract those muscles and then release them. Once the muscles are relaxed, make a mental note if you feel anything. Pain, tension, relief, numbness, etc. After you have gathered the information, continue to work your way down your body using the diagram below, from your head down to your feet. When you are finished, circle the areas where you felt a sensation and describe the feeling.

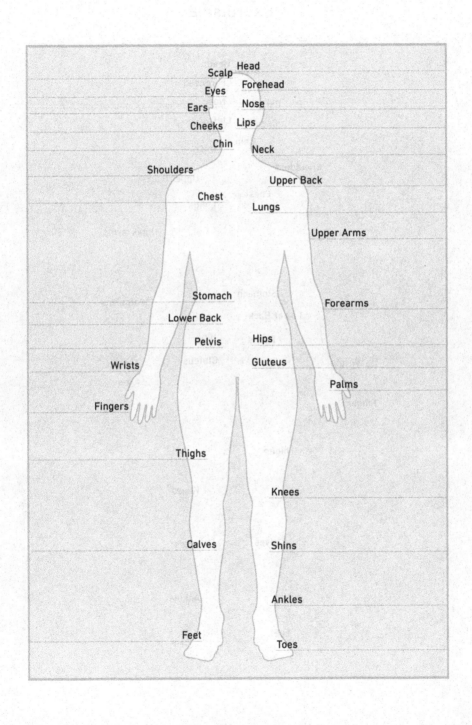

Exercise 2

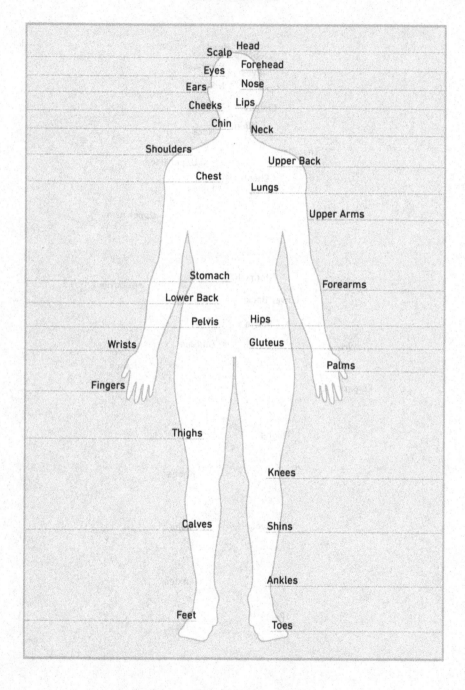

Look over your diagram above. If you feel tension or fatigue in any part of your body, lie back down and try to sink into a relaxed state. We want to send a rejuvenating breath to the places that need a little love. If your feet feel tired and painful, take a deep breath in through your nose for a count of three. Hold your breath for a moment when you get to three. Then, on an exhale, imagine sending the breath down to the area that feels pain. As you do this, repeat the following phrase three times: "My feet feel light." The goal here is to change the sensation to get that body part to relax. Take another deep breath, send the exhale breath down to your feet, and repeat the following phrase three times: "My feet feel fresh." Work your way through each area that feels tense or painful. When you're done, make a note about how you feel now.

Exercise 3

Do this on your next run. After about a mile, begin to mentally scan your body, starting at your toes. Check in with them: "Toes, how are you feeling?" Note any issues. Is there a body part that feels heavy, tired, tense, or achy? If so, take a long inhale and send the long exhale to the fatigued area. Try to repeat the phrases: "My _____ feels light" and "My _____ feels fresh." For example, if you have a side stitch, take a breath in, and then on the exhale, send the breath down to where the pain is and repeat, "My side feels light," in your head three times. Then say, "My side feels fresh," in your head three times. When you're done with your run, go through the diagram below, noting any issues, what you did to try to fix them, what worked, and what didn't work.

Try to repeat this every day for a week. Once you figure out what works best for your body, the scans don't have to be as formal, though I do recommend doing both a resting and a running scan at least weekly while in training. You might begin to notice patterns. And you might be able to pick up on potential injuries—and seek strategies to heal before they take you out. As you start to communicate with your body through breath and feel, you can remedy tension on the fly.

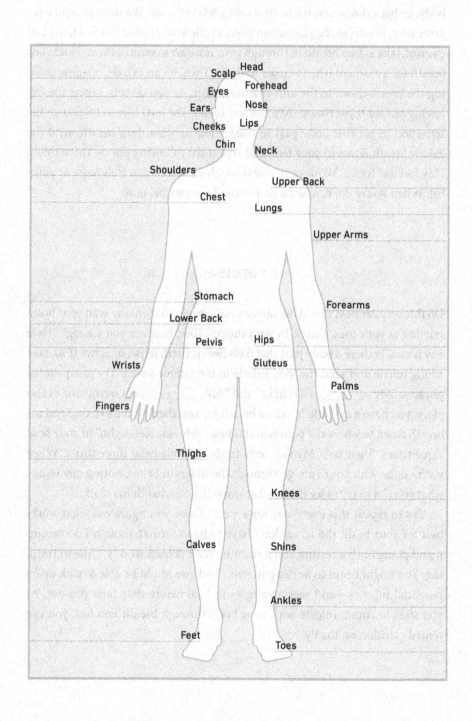

CONNECT THE BRAIN AND BODY

Most marathoners know how much mental effort is required in running. It's a thinking sport, even though there isn't a heckuva lot of strategy. That dichotomy can create issues. "What can hinder a race is our mind getting in our way," says Hillary Israelsen, a sports psychologist at HeadStrong Consulting. That might sound counterintuitive—but really it's our thinking ego that often chatters so much that it increases self-doubt or anxiety, or even just uses a bunch of energy that you could better spend getting through a three-to-six-hour race.

All the negative-thinking traps that could potentially damage your running are a product of your internal self getting all judgy. Here's the thing: you know how to run. Your body knows how it wants to feel when it runs. Heck, if you've been running for a year or so, you probably know what pace you're running without looking at your watch. Advanced runners, you know how fast you're running, but I bet you feel like you need to know the exact numbers. You don't.

One of the greatest gifts you can give yourself is running free. If you run by feel instead of depending on a constant stream of data, I can guarantee that you will succeed in your training. Instead of letting your internal self—the one who is distracted by life, or the one who feels the need to be perfect, or the one who always thinks it is not good enough—instead of letting that person control your running, let your body take over. Tell the ego to be quiet and let you do your thing. Don't analyze your running—that is the critical self trying to interfere. All this does is slow you down. Just go out, listen to your breath, and get grounded in the run.

When your thinking mind is out of the way and you're really grounded in your run, you're able to enter the zone. You've probably heard of this concept of the zone. Or flow state. Or whatever buzzword you want to throw out there to describe that state of ecstasy when you are so fully in your body doing something that the rest of the world melts away. Athletes at any level can all name a time when their body took over completely. Some athletes have even reported blacking out during this state or feeling like they were dreaming. It's a kind of out-of-body experience that allows for absolute peak performance because the ego disappears.

Hillary Israelsen tells me that with a lot of practice, you can experience that brilliant state more often. "You can't force flow," she says. "But the more you build your mental game, the more likely you are to achieve it in practice or competition. And the mental tools used in a variety of situations will give you the confidence to know that if flow isn't happening that day, you can still create the success you are looking for."

Mental training will open up communication between your conscious mind and physical being. At the end of the day, we want our mind to be sending out signals that say, "Hey, body, I trust you. I'm not going to waste your time chatting back here. I'm just going to shut up and enjoy the ride."

But that's easier said than done, right? How do we get our minds to get out of the way? My brain has been a chronic issue in my performance. That's why I called Hillary in the first place. The good thing is, there are a lot of strategies to help combat the thinking mind. Below are the strategies that I find most effective.

TRUST-YOUR-BODY TEST

Here's a super simple test. Stand on one foot for thirty seconds, then switch feet. If you can't do this, practice. Believe it or not, balance is important to running.

Once you're able to do this with ease, you can take the next test. Close your eyes and stand on one foot. Try to hold for thirty seconds. Repeat on the other foot.

If you can do this without an issue, then that's great. First, your balance is good! Yay! Second, your brain is likely letting your body do the work for you without trying to control everything.

If it was tough for you to maintain your balance with your eyes closed, try this before you close your eyes: remind your mind that your body is in one place and it is not moving. Sometimes just communicating with your body about what to do is enough to stop all that wobbling around. Your mind is very strong, and if your mind thinks your body is capable of handling a task, your body will do it.

Standing on one foot with your eyes closed is an incredible exercise. If it's simple for you, try to exceed the thirty seconds and record your best effort. If you can't make it to thirty seconds, then jot down how long you can hold it for. Practice every day. I do it while I'm brushing my teeth with my electronic toothbrush, holding thirty seconds four times.

INTRODUCTION TO IMAGERY

You've likely heard about using imagery techniques to improve sports performance, and for good reason. In many cases, it works—but only if it's done correctly. Too many of us are merely imagining a race situation every once in a while and then relying on that one image. Sure, thinking about crossing the finish line when you're at the start is certainly motivational, but it's not what sports psychologists would consider a true imagery practice. Now, skeptics might be thinking, "Can I really think my way to a faster time?" Hillary Israelsen says that the practice helps flip the switch to get into the zone. You can reap the full benefits of imagery practice if you start out by (1) establishing a consistent, daily routine and (2) getting all your senses involved.

First, it's important to note that imagery is not merely imagining or visualizing something. You want to build up the experience so that it is completely immersive. By the time you've been practicing for a month or so, you might be able to engage all five senses, but this is an exercise for your mind, and to build strength, you have to start light.

Get comfortable in a seated position or lying down. Close your eyes and picture yourself the moment before you begin to run. Pick a setting that's familiar—a road you always run on, or the end of your driveway where you begin your run. The more specific you can be, the better. Spend a few moments looking around and silently name a few things you see. Once you're oriented, picture yourself beginning to move. Start a slow run. Try to maintain this focus for twenty seconds.

When you open your eyes, I want you to remember if you were in the first-person perspective (looking at the world around you through your own eyes) or if you were in the third person (looking at yourself) as you ran. Both perspectives are fine for right now. If you can, try to switch between them every other day. But in these early stages of imagery practice, you can go with whatever perspective is most comfortable.

Pick a time of day to dedicate to a daily imagery practice. Hillary says that if maintaining twenty seconds of focus is too easy, you should increase the time to forty seconds. Practice that until you can sustain the perspective with ease. The key is to keep a solid image and then increase the time as your ability grows.

For the first week, focus on setting the scene. You are simply to imagine yourself running, relaxed, and notice what you see. Watch what happens as an active observer on your run.

The next week, add another sense. For me, the easiest one to incorporate is sound. I will open my ears and imagine birdcalls and then the sound of my own feet on the pavement. You might hear your breath.

Each week add a new sense. Smell is an amazing tool for memory, so you might want to add scents that represent good runs. Maybe it's fresh-cut grass, or a body of water you pass on your run, or the smell of the heat radiating off the pavement. Taste then might stem from what you're smelling. Or you might be able to detect the dryness in your mouth and the first sip of water. All of this will lead up to touch—you might be able to focus on the feeling of your feet rebounding off the ground, your arms as they gently sway against your sides, your heart pumping, your hot blood coursing through your extremities, and your breath rising and falling.

By employing all your senses and really feeling the bodily sensations, you can create a running scenario that is pleasant and gratifying. Be aware of what's around you, feel yourself in the moment, and let your body do the work. The more you work on this imagery, the more your active mind will let go and allow your body to do its thing when you're really out on the roads.

The way imagery works and why it is effective is a pretty interesting phenomenon. When we plan and execute a movement or skill, we use various neural networks in our brains. I like to think of them as information highways with thoughts zooming around to make our bodies act how we want them to. When researchers took a look at people's brains when they were using imagery and when they were engaged in the skill or activity that they used the imagery for, the same areas lit up. There's an overlap in neural networks where imagery and performance live! So basically, the same places in our minds are active when we're physically performing and when we're using imagery.

It follows that your brain and body will benefit from imagery, because you can essentially create a perfect training and racing scenario. This might help you run at your best without worry because you've trained those neural networks. They will activate more accurately and readily during the actual performance.

PERSPECTIVES

When you're first starting your imagery journey, feel free to use whatever perspective feels more comfortable and gets you most immersed in the scene. But as you progress and want to advance even further, you can start to choose your point of view based on your goals.

If you want to create a moment when you are experiencing the run and seeing things as you would see them during a workout, then go internal and view the world from a first-person point of view. Using this method is great for preparedness and confidence. Let's say, for example, your training plan calls for a track workout. Maybe it's a tough one, like 8 x 800, and you're doubting your ability to get through the whole thing. This scenario would be a perfect time to create an image in the first person, running the last eight hundred. By feeling yourself do it internally, your mind and body will be primed to conquer the workout.

The first-person POV can work in specific areas of improvement as well. Maybe you want to focus on a faster foot turnover, which is to say, you want your feet to leave the ground at a faster rate per stride. Turning inward is a good option to home in on the kinesthetic imagery, meaning you can use this to feel a sensation in your feet and legs as well as gather external tactile information (the feet making contact with the ground).

If you want to work on your form, or get a sense of a course, or get an aerial view of a particular area of concern (like a hill that always gets you), then adopting the position of an observer can be very beneficial. In terms of body positioning, picking a vantage point outside yourself can help you "try on" the right form. Third-person POV allows you to see information that would not be available from the first-person perspective. It will show your body what it should look like and then lock the image into memory. If you want to work on quickening your turnover, you can watch yourself externally and visualize yourself running your desired cadence with confidence. How do you know the proper form to try on? Try watching your favorite elite runner on YouTube right before you start your visualization.

An aerial view can help diminish anxiety, fatigue, or any negative feelings or emotions you may have developed toward certain parts of your training. It could be something physical, like a hill or a long curve. Or it could be the last half mile of a tempo run or mile sixteen of a long run. Imagining the scenario of yourself in motion—pumping your legs, breathing with ease, looking strong—can bolster your confidence when faced with whatever you perceive as your challenge.

Choosing what to focus on in your imagery sessions depends on timing and the desired effect. Right now, we want to cultivate the feeling of a determined state of mind for training. You might also pick one skill to improve, like mastering a smooth stride or calm breathing.

In the early sessions of imagery work, a little bit of note taking can help you focus. Before an imagery session, write down what you want to see, hear, smell, taste, and feel. Afterward, record what perspective you used and what senses you successfully incorporated into your session. Finally, write down how you feel emotionally after the session.

BREATHE RIGHT

Too often runners think about what our limbs are doing and neglect what could arguably be the most important part of our sport. Your breath plays a vital role in getting you to the finish line, and it's possible, with a little practice, to make it work for you.

Have you ever had the experience of another runner coming up behind you wheezing and grunting and coughing? When I notice someone running like this, it's clear to me that they won't be able to sustain their current pace for very long. How do I know this? Because their breath is out of control.

Being able to use your breath does amazing things for your mental stamina, concentration, and overall running ability. When we talk about our easy runs, many coaches and experts use the talk test. Are you running at a pace that allows you to carry on a conversation? It's a good baseline, and if I'm running alone, I try to sing (quietly, I swear) to see if I'm doing things right. But I never could master the talk-test pace until I learned how to get my breath under control.

That's right. Full confession: I used to be one of those annoying, gasping-for-air, about-to-keel-over-on-the-trail type of runners. For my first marathon, I was fortunate enough to train with the legendary running coach and Olympic Trials qualifier Budd Coates, who literally wrote the book on breathing while running. It's called *Running on Air*, and it really demonstrates the power of your breath.

Coates uses a simple formula to help you match your steps to your breath. For slow easy runs, he says to use 3:2. This means you inhale for three steps, then exhale for the next two steps. So basically, you would breathe your first breath in as your right foot hits the ground, then another inhale for left, then inhale right, exhale left, exhale right. This was revolutionary for me. Suddenly, I was breathing with control and ease. Coates says that this pattern will prevent overstriding because you are forced to match your steps with your cardiovascular ability. Overstriding, or taking too big of a step while running, can cause your muscles to get tired too quickly and is a recipe for injury.

Now let's say you want to pick up the pace. Switch it to a 2:1 pattern. Right foot inhale, left inhale, right exhale, left inhale, right inhale, left exhale. This method allows you to quicken your stride but won't let you set yourself on fire when you're trying to run.

Now, just because your breathing is controlled, it doesn't mean running will be without huffing and puffing. During easy runs, ragged breathing is your first indication that you should slow down. To slow down, I like to take twenty walking steps. While walking, I take very deep inhales through my nose and then release with open-mouth exhales. Then I resume running. In your speedier workouts, you might feel your breath get a bit out of control. That's OK if you're nearing the end of a repeat and have a chance to recover within ten seconds. But if you're starting out breathing haphazardly, chances are you're going too fast.

Breath work also lets your mind relax. Your ego self—the one who might be trying to tell you that you're running too slow or too fast—is given a distraction. She has to count and breathe. Meanwhile, the runner you're meant to be takes over. It's like a moving meditation that keeps you very tuned in and focused but launches you into a state above the conscious self.

SELF-COMPASSION

You can do a million body scans and imagery sessions and breathe like an Olympian, but if you aren't kind to yourself in a fundamental way, your mind will inevitably hold you back from reaching your goals. So many of us speak negatively to ourselves—and sometimes we don't even know we're doing it.

Hillary Israelsen says that she often has to wake women up and make them see that there are consequences of their negativity. "The first thing is getting them to become aware of when they are using negative self-talk and the effect it is having on their performance," she says.

Think about it. Do you beat yourself up if you feel slow on a particular day? What do you tell yourself when you miss a run? Are you being nice to the image you see in the mirror?

I bring this up because it's an issue that tripped me up on many a training cycle. I never used to think that I was beating myself up. I thought that I was making myself better, striving for all my goals, and being tough. Little did I know that this strange alter ego who was obsessed with perfection was actually berating the perfectly fine, perfectly capable runner inside me. I first realized the flaw in my thought processes when I announced, after a particularly grueling 5K, "I am two minutes off my best time. I should be able to run faster. I am so out of shape. I better start doing speed work, like, tomorrow."

A wonderful running buddy who happens to be a running coach looked at me and said, "Would you speak to anyone else that way? Is that what you would say to an athlete after a race if you were their coach?"

Obviously not. My friend suggested I spend a week noticing what other nasty things I was saying inside my own head. She told me to try to rephrase whatever evil I was spewing in a way that I would speak to a close friend or my younger, five-year-old self. It seemed silly at first, but after a week I noticed that the negative self-talk was a bad habit.

I asked Hillary for her professional opinion and what she advises her clients to do. She underscored that developing grit in running performance does not mean speaking negatively to yourself. Here's what Hillary recommends.

Thought Stopping

This means you visualize a stop sign or say the word *stop* to get the string of negative thoughts to stop. Once you have stopped the negative thoughts, you have to replace them immediately or they will come back. Make this new thought an "I am" statement that is something you are working toward achieving. Some good examples are "I am capable" or "I am confident" or "I am improving each day." It must be a solid "I am" statement; otherwise doubt will sneak in.

Write five "I am" statements:

1. I am_____

2. I am_____

3. I am_____

4. I am_____

5. I am_____

Refocus

Instead of thinking about the worst-case scenario or what you don't want to happen, think about the best possible outcome. Instead of saying, "Don't slow down" or "What if I don't hit my paces?" focus on something you want to happen. Try "I'm feeling speedy" and "I'm going to nail my paces" or "Today is my day."

Reframe

When the negative self-talk comes into your brain, turn it into something positive. Instead of "I am so tired, my legs feel like concrete," reframe to "My legs feel like concrete because I have run twenty miles. That's a lot of miles. I know these legs can get me to the end."

Erase *Should*

Get the word *should* out of your vocabulary and practice some self-compassion. If you think, "I should've run farther," try "I ran for a really long time, and I'm only going to get stronger." If after a missed run, you think, "I should've run today. I can't believe I skipped it," try "I'll get the next run in. One session won't make or break the race" or "I gave my body a break and maybe that's just what it needed."

If you're slightly more neurotic than the average cat and obsess about your training plan, pace, and general performance (raises hand), or you notice increased anxiety while you're training, look for a sports psychologist to lean on. For example, if you ever feel like crying because of a less-than-ideal time, a therapist can really help. If you show up to the track and feel so anxious that your breathing is out of control and your legs feel heavy, a professional will give you ways to cope. They can help you identify the root cause of these thoughts and guide you in making positive thinking a habit. Of course, I know not all of us have the resources to spend on our mental health. In an ideal world, I would say that you have to prioritize this. But in the real world, know that I know you are trying your best. I would also recommend the app Youper, which has helped me tremendously.

While missing a training day or slowing your pace will not ruin your running career, a bad habit of negativity could very well derail you. Sometimes the rigidity, exhaustion, and demands of marathon training can exacerbate thinking distortions. Think about it as you would an injury: get it checked out, do some prehab and rehab, and know that this little extra self-care will make you a better runner.

CHAPTER 8

FEED YOUR MACHINE

W hen it comes to runners not performing at their peak, not eating enough and not eating well are too often the culprits. Our active bodies need the right combination of foods and fluids to get us through our marathon journey. The good news is that this problem has a solution, though it may take some trial and error to find what works for you. The key is finding a solution that is simple, implementing changes slowly, and creating a sustainable nutrition plan that doesn't feel oppressive. Believe me, I understand the need for things to be simple and sustainable when it comes to eating.

For as long as I can remember, I've had a strange relationship with food. I think *dysfunctional* would be an overstatement, but *off* is probably the best way to describe it. When I first devoted my life to running and health, I seesawed between restricting calories and declaring war on diets. Some weeks I would eat only greens and fruits, then pivot to an all-orange diet consisting primarily of cheese puffs and Creamsicles. My mind-set went back and forth between the need to "be healthy" and the need to tell the fad-diet industrial complex to shove it. I felt confusion, guilt, shame, elation—all these extreme emotions at various mealtimes.

I didn't, however, feel satisfied or strong. It wasn't until I met Heather Mayer Irvine, a nutrition scientist and former nutrition editor for *Runner's World* magazine, that I realized my thinking about food was downright irrational. When we were coworkers and had neighboring offices, Heather witnessed my daily ritual of skipping lunch, then eating several protein bars at 3:00 p.m., then stuffing my face with chips or whatever I could find around the office at 4:00 p.m. On days when I was being "healthy," she saw me toting around celery sticks, a protein shake, and four apples. These extremes, she let me know, were not good for running, let alone marathon training. The way to think about eating or diet or whatever you want to call it was to recognize that what you consume is the energy you have to burn. Your food is fuel.

I realized that I was either running on empty or filling myself with crappy low-grade sludge gas. Shifting my mind-set, keeping a consistent eating schedule, and making an effort to fill my diet with good stuff was a process. But once I started to feel more energetic, I knew this was a pivotal piece of my training regimen. I tell you about this only because I know I am not alone. Many female runners report having disordered eating—that includes anorexia, bulimia, and binge eating disorder. On a lesser extreme, every nutritionist I talked to when researching this chapter told me that the number one issue in nutrition for female marathoners is not eating enough calories.

When we are troubleshooting for problems in training, the first question you need to ask yourself is "Am I eating enough?" The second: "Am I eating the right foods?"

So what does that mean exactly? It would be really easy for me to tell you that you need to consume X number of calories for every mile run. Some articles and books might give you a number. But before I impose rules on you, I think it's necessary to acknowledge that when it comes to fueling, every runner and body is different. A lot of factors go into how many calories to consume and what foods to eat, including your dietary restrictions, your height, your current weight, and your lifestyle. If you are someone who struggles with fatigue in training or who feels they've hit a running plateau or who is steadfast about losing pounds while training, the best gift you can give yourself is an appointment with a nutritionist or dietician. Of course, not everyone is able to pay for an individual plan, so use this chapter as a foundation for tweaks you can make in your nutrition.

If eating enough or eating good food is something you struggle with, I want you to grab a notebook and try to keep a record of your meals. Do not use this to obsessively count calories. Instead, make lists of what you eat, when you eat it, how you feel on your run, and how you feel overall.

THE BASICS

The key to keeping your energy stores up is to maintain balance and variety. In terms of what to eat, studies show that runners should eat the same way that's advised for everyone else, and that is 50 to 60 percent healthy carbohydrates, 15 to 20 percent protein, and 15 to 20 percent healthy fats.

Each of these categories serve a different purpose.

Carbohydrates

Think of carbs as your star power source. We need them for our brains and bodies to work. When carbs are digested, they are broken down into smaller sugar molecules called glucose, which is then stored as usable fuel in the liver and muscles. Carbohydrates delay fatigue and aid in muscle repair, helping protein do its job. Some healthy carbohydrates include:

- Quinoa
- Potatoes
- Beans
- Beets
- Oatmeal
- Whole wheat wraps
- Sprouted-grain bread
- Brown rice
- All fruits
- Literally any vegetable

Protein

Protein is made up of amino acids, which are essential to building and repairing muscles. There is actually a pretty great calculation to figure out how much protein you need.

I am . . .	I work out . . .	My workout duration is . . .	Daily protein needs
Active	4–5 days per week	Averaging 30–50 minutes per session	0.5 grams of protein per pound of body weight
Super active	5–6 days per week	Averaging 50 minutes or more per session	0.75 grams of protein per pound of body weight

You have to remember, of course, that this number might change if you work a physically strenuous job. It might need to change if you went from sedentary to active fairly quickly. You can use an online calculator to try to figure out your needs. You can also talk to a registered dietician. No matter what, add the following to your shopping list, because these healthy foods are go-tos for runners. (Vegetarians, just ignore the meat and fish.) Healthy proteins include:

- Greek yogurt
- Cottage cheese
- Chicken
- Turkey
- Salmon
- Eggs
- Almonds
- Milk
- Tuna
- Whey protein isolate

Fats

Remember how we spent the last two decades demonizing fats? Yeah, whoops. Consuming a moderate amount of good fats allows the body to process nutrients efficiently and gives it the ability to absorb vitamins A, D, E, and K. Plus, it supplies athletes with long-lasting energy. Good fats include:

- Avocados
- Eggs
- Salmon
- Almonds
- Chia seeds
- Olive oil
- Nut butters

The difference between athletes and everyone else is the quantity we need to eat. Simply put, runners need calories! It's also important to keep in mind that as your training volume and intensity change throughout the year, the amount you eat should correspond. Many professional athletes will consume more than three thousand calories per day at the peak of their training. Based on your intensity, volume, and body type, you might need to match or exceed that number.

NO FOOD IS EVIL

I don't need to spell out the foods that won't benefit your training. Sure, we can aspire to cut down on our soda intake and reduce our french fry consumption. You might feel powerless against the call of these highly addictive foods and ashamed that they are what you crave the most. Don't! This is common, even for a great number of athletes. The best part is, you don't have to listen to the headlines that tell you how hard it is to quit sugar. You don't have to quit sugar at all, in fact. You just won't need it or crave it anymore if you make a few small daily changes.

Body composition expert Dez McQueen says that whenever she has an athlete who is a sugar fiend or dependent on processed foods, she takes a slow and multipronged approach to help them get over the addiction. First, when it comes to junk foods—especially sugar—cold turkey is not the best method. She says to make small tweaks, like switching from a sugary breakfast cereal to oatmeal with nuts, fruit, and a teaspoon of honey. Making that change might be enough for a week. Next she will help the client tackle added sugars that are lurking in their lunch, then their dinner, and so on.

Often our cravings for processed foods are both physical and emotional. We think about treats as rewards. You know how I asked you at the beginning of this chapter to track your meals? Now is the time to pay attention to the emotions tied to what you're eating and when you're eating it. If I fry up an egg in the morning and feel no type of way, that seems like a very neutral interaction with food. But if I do my run in the evening, come home, eat dinner, feel fine but tired and maybe a little stressed from the day, and think, "I need something to help me feel satisfied," and then go into the freezer and dig around for a pint of ice cream, then . . . back up the train. There is a lot going on right there! When I think of ice cream, I'm making the following associations: it will make me feel better, it will help me relax, I earned it. But guess what? The ice cream doesn't have the power to do any of those things! Your mind does, though.

By interrupting these associations (many of which have been programmed into us since the time we were children) we can take back control. Instead of depriving ourselves of the ice cream because we've deemed it bad and unhealthy, we can use our brains to manage stress, congratulate ourselves for our efforts, and find other coping methods to help us after a long day. We will not internalize the lack of dessert as a sort of punishment. Instead, by eating the fuel that will make us feel and perform great, we will feel as though we are treating our bodies well.

Here's a step-by-step guide to stopping a craving in its tracks:

> The craving: Ice cream
> The thought: I am finally finished with work after a long day. Ice cream will make me relax.

The feeling: Stress

The detective work: Why am I stressed?

The answer: My to-do list is never-ending; I want everything to be
   perfect.

The alternative thought: It is fine to be stressed. Is there something
   else that can help this feeling?

The action: Write down the three most pressing items on the to-do
   list and put it away. Boil water for tea.

The new thought: This tea is soothing. Everything will get done. I
   am proud for calming myself down.

Staying hydrated while weaning off sugar or processed foods will help ease discomfort. If you make small adjustments and revamp your diet mindfully, your withdrawal symptoms will be so mild, you will hardly feel them at all. Having done this myself, I guarantee this to be true!

Finally, there's no need to blacklist foods. Simply recognize that they won't convert into a clean fuel that will improve performance. Then resolve to enjoy (and I mean really, mindfully, take the time to enjoy) these treats in moderation.

TIMING

Many nutritionists agree that in addition to three great meals each day, runners should graze. Snacking on the right foods will help your body keep up with the energy expenditure happening in your training and maintain your blood sugar levels. But grazing doesn't work for everyone—especially if you are someone who is busy and needs structure (or doesn't have enough teeny Tupperware to last you every day).

Heather Caplan, a dietician for Lift Run Perform, makes a great case for keeping a firm eating schedule. "Many people don't realize that the adrenaline produced when you run can actually act as an appetite suppressant," she says. "Often runners don't even realize they are skipping precious calories that they desperately need. Just because you don't feel hungry doesn't mean you aren't hungry. It may just mean that your body is all hopped up on endorphins."

Caplan recommends getting some food in your system about every two hours. It doesn't have to be special protein muffins made just for runners. It can be a banana and some almonds. You could grab a package of those premade peanut butter and jelly sandwiches with the crusts cut off from the freezer aisle. In any case, eat at evenly spaced intervals, because at some point (four hours for most people) your runner's high will wear off and you will be ravenous and unable to meet the energy needs for your body to build and repair muscle.

Before and after your runs are pivotal eating times. Carbs are your power, your energy, your prerun fuel. Ensure that you get a small meal, complete with carbs, protein, and fat, about three to four hours before your workout for the day. One or two hours beforehand, snack on something small, maybe crackers or an apple. I've listed some additional ideas below.

Immediately following your run, you must turn your attention to replacing the fluids you've lost through sweat and urine. That means hydrating with water but also getting something more substantial, meaning electrolytes, to help your body absorb the liquid. More on this below in the hydration section.

In terms of food, you need to consume something within forty minutes of your workout to replenish your glycogen stores. Getting some easily digestible carbs in your system ASAP will aid in the repair of the muscles you wore down. That means a stronger you! Add a little protein, and you will be in recovery heaven. Your postworkout fuel doesn't need to be anything fancy or gourmet. It could actually be a low-sugar protein drink. Or it could be a baked potato topped with Greek yogurt. At the very least, grab a sports drink like Gatorade and a protein bar. Consuming a little sugar won't kill you and is better than not eating anything at all.

Preworkout Food Ideas

Consume 1–2 hours before your workout

Apple and nut butter
Oatmeal with berries

Hard-boiled egg and whole wheat crackers

Yogurt topped with nuts and fruit

Banana and a protein bar

Ezekiel bread with sliced turkey and cheese

Postworkout Food Ideas

Consume immediately after your workout

Chocolate milk

Protein drink and banana

Cottage cheese with granola and berries

Consume within three hours after your workout

Eggs with spinach and toast

Oatmeal topped with apples, nuts, honey, and
cinnamon

Grilled chicken, avocado, and brown rice

Salmon with quinoa and broccoli

HYDRATING

Water and electrolytes act as carriers of oxygen in your body, maintaining a stable blood pressure and heart rate. They lubricate joints, ensure that your muscles are functional (and not cramping), and help your body temperature stay level by giving your body something to sweat out. So when you deprive yourself of water and electrolytes, your system goes haywire. If you ever measure your pulse rate on a day when you aren't hydrated, you'll notice that it's higher, which will cause general fatigue and a decrease in performance.

Signs you need more fluids

Dark yellow pee
Low urine output
Muscle cramps
High heart rate
High body temperature
Low sweat output

Did you know that you can lose four pounds of water when you run? That's a lot of water. Surely if you didn't replace that, you'd feel miserable. But many runners are walking around depleted and not even knowing why. The golden rule of drinking eight ounces eight times a day is a fine baseline, but there is a little more to it than that.

You can do the pee test as a nonscientific way to measure your levels. Basically, check the color of your pee—if it's pale yellow, you're okay. If it's dark yellow or orange, you need more water! If it is clear, you might be too hydrated. Some elite runners will weigh themselves before and after runs to know exactly how much water weight was lost in a workout and then attempt to consume what was lost within four hours postrun. If you want to try this method, drink twenty-four ounces of fluid for every pound lost.

It's important, though, to keep your body hydrated throughout the day and during your run. Too many of us don't hydrate as we run, even though that's the easiest way to keep our bodies from losing fluids. Just as you train your muscles, you need to train yourself to drink. If you're guilty of skimping on hydration, then start slow. Bring a water bottle with you even on your shorter runs. That will get you used to carrying whatever vessel you choose. If you're out for a three-miler, take a sip once, just to try it. Slowly work your way up. Make sure you are sipping—chugging will cause that terrible glugging feeling in your belly. Hydration needs on long runs and race days will vary depending on the weather. If you're sweating more, you will need more fluids. Ideally, you will take in small amounts of liquid before you're parched. Hydrating shouldn't be rocket science. If your mouth starts to get dry, drink something. If you feel thirsty, drink something. Let your thirst be your guide.

You could be on the other end of the spectrum and drowning your muscles without realizing it. I see many runners aimlessly filling up their water bottles over and over again throughout the day and wondering why they feel tired and bloated. Body fluids consist primarily of water and electrolytes such as salt and smaller amounts of potassium, and you need to replace both. When you drink too much water, you're throwing that water and electrolyte balance off. That doesn't mean you have to invest in specialty water or drink a sports drink, though both of those are fine options. One nutritionist who worked with me to reduce my overhydrating problem told me to sprinkle about an eighth of a teaspoon of mineral salt in four of my daily eight-ounce glasses.

Hydration Plan

Water and a pinch of salt
Water and a splash of fruit juice
Pickle juice
Sports drinks

FUEL YOUR LONG RUN

It wasn't until recently that exercise scientists realized that proper fueling could increase a runner's performance by up to 20 percent. And back in the days when the only people running marathons were men, the common thought was that one should not eat anything at all during runs. Some of these fools didn't even consume water. Welp, let's not do that.

During your long runs, not only do you need to hydrate, but you need to fuel as well. The golden rule is that if you are going to do a run that is longer than ninety minutes, you should be consuming some sort of calories along the way. There's a plethora of easy, on-the-go gels and candies that runners use.

There are also a few different techniques to get those calories in. Traditionalists will tell you that the ideal amount of carbohydrates to consume is fifteen grams every fifteen minutes. That could also translate to sixty grams per hour. Too many runners use the hour mark as a rule of thumb and just shove a bunch of glucose and fructose into their mouths at the sixty-minute mark. Don't wait that long. Eat something fifteen or thirty minutes into the run.

Waiting for five or six miles and then introducing a whole bunch of sugar into your system will likely backfire and cause some unwanted blood sugar fluctuations and GI issues. Most gels and gummies have about twenty-five grams of carbs in them, so you could eat two of those packets every thirty minutes plus sip some sports drink along the way. No matter if you're drinking sports drinks or plain water, you should take a sip every time you eat.

Lately, some brave marathoners have been using the ultramarathoner model of fueling. If you've never seen a water and fuel station at one of these races, I encourage you to go check it out. The spread at these things makes running 50K or more very tempting. I'm talking gummy bears, Swedish fish, pretzels, sandwiches, breakfast pastries, sodas, cookies. Yeah, when you're running that many miles, you need to graze for the entire race to keep you going. I recently spoke to a marathoner who bucked the traditional fueling strategies and decided to nibble on various candies, crackers, and even some rice balls throughout her training and race. She swears she felt stronger. She had historically experienced GI distress and thought that it might have been because her stomach shut down when it wasn't being used. So she tried the approach of eating something small every mile. Will this work for everyone? No. Many of us would be sick as heck and need a porta-potty by mile three. But it worked for her because she experimented long before race day.

The main takeaway is this: practice what, how, and when you take in calories. When something works, write down exactly what you did and try to replicate it.

On-the-Go Fuel Options

Gels

Gummies

Jelly beans
Honey
Maple syrup
Sports drinks
Dried fruits

RECOVER

Don't skimp on calories just because you aren't running or training on your rest day. It's not scientifically proven that comforting, soothing foods on recovery days will add to your gains, but it is proven that getting enough protein will! I like to make sure my rest-day meals are both protein packed and scrumptious. I can guarantee that this is the winning combination to feel amazing physically and mentally. I make these meals part of my self-care routine and take the time to fully experience every bite.

On days following long runs, you might feel ravenous. That endless hunger is your body telling your brain that your energy stores are depleted. You know how dieticians tell you not to go grocery shopping hungry? Trying to decide what to eat the day after a long run is essentially the same thing. You cannot trust your hungry brain to make good decisions. I know from experience—if the right food isn't already in my house, I will reach for easy solutions like doughnuts and bags of chips. Making a plan the day before will help ensure that you get the proper nutrients.

THE WEIGHT-LOSS TRAP

Many women use the marathon as a means to achieve their extrinsic goal of weight loss. When I asked Heather Caplan about this trend, she noted that this desire is totally understandable. "It's shoved down our throats," she says. "The relationship between running and weight loss is something generated by the media, but nobody talks about how your body might change in the course of marathon training in such a way that you actually gain weight. Would that matter if you are healthier, or would that be a devastating outcome? That's important to determine before setting that goal."

I hope that those of you who are reading this will refer back to chapter 1 and consider reframing the weight-loss goal to be more than a number on a scale.

Why? Well, because that number does not reflect your progress. In the course of marathon training, your weight will fluctuate. You might retain water one day or plateau because your body is desperately clinging to what it perceives as an energy source. You know that weight gain Caplan is talking about? That gain could be all muscle. While it's true that a lighter runner is a swifter runner, that works only if your body is in balance and has enough muscle to carry it forward. You shouldn't try to lose weight at the risk of losing muscle. See how paying attention to the scale could actually cause more harm than good?

A lot of us have spent our whole lives reading about diets and how best to keep our figures. The diet industry has fed into our paranoias, and I want you to free yourself from its shackles! Trying to be the healthiest version of yourself is a better motivator. When you feel like being lighter fits into that plan, I invite you to think about it as balancing your body composition—not losing pounds. When you look at your weight and BMI exclusively, all you're doing is comparing how heavy you are with a standard that might not fit your individual goals. On the other hand, body composition measures your muscle-to-fat ratio and takes your bones and water weight into account too. Many personal trainers, nutritionists, doctors, and body composition experts can help you in measuring your body fat percentage, which is a number that will offer insights into your total body composition.

A FEW FINAL WORDS

Unless your doctor tells you otherwise, most of your vitamins will come from food. You don't need to invest in special vitamins or mixtures or magic potions made specifically for runners. We can all try to make our diets healthier, but aim for progress, not perfection. Add the foods in this chapter to your shopping list and see what makes you feel best. If something feels amiss, consult an expert. But really, keep it simple: Eat for energy. When you want to treat yourself, do so in moderation. If you feel tired, recall what you've consumed and check if it is high quality and the right quantity. This should be the first step in troubleshooting for fatigue.

In the process of training for a marathon, you will be hungry a lot and you will need to eat—sometimes a lot. I guarantee that you will crave a wide variety of foods. But I can also guarantee that something magical happens. As you log more miles and focus on your goals, your subconscious mind will tune in and fall in line. By week three, your brain will send signals demanding fresh, whole foods. All you have to do is trust yourself.

CHAPTER 9

IN-SEASON TRAINING

4 months

Goals: Race-specific training, increase mileage and intensity, muscle maintenance

Welcome, my friend, to in-season training. At this point, you have worked so hard, learned about yourself, and picked a race. Now that you are here, it's time to start thinking about race day. Your mileage and speed training will be more intense and gradually increase. By the end of the third month and the beginning of the fourth month of in-season training, you will be shocked by how much you're able to handle. I mean, we're talking forty-mile weeks! Remember when you were only running ten-mile weeks? Can you believe how far you've come?

You've built strength and mileage, got your brain right, and have some basic nutrition skills down. But there are a few more tips and tricks to learn as you go through the next sixteen weeks. First, there is a whole new strength training regimen for you to master. Second, there is a delightful menu of workouts meant to target speed and endurance in an upcoming section called "Kick Your Own Butt." I don't mean to get your hopes too high, but these workouts are *super* fun. Third, I will empower you to know when you are working hard and grinding throughout in-season training and when you are overdoing it.

Erica Coviello's Beginner In-Season Training Plan

Week	Monday	Tuesday	Wednesday
1	•Strength A + C •Easy run 3 miles	•Low-impact cross-train	•Strength B + C •Easy run 4 miles
2	•Strength B + C •Easy run 4 miles	•Low-impact cross-train	•Strength A + C •Easy run 4 miles
3	•Strength A + C •Easy run 4 miles	•Low-impact cross-train	•Strength B + C •Easy run 5 miles
4	•Strength B + C •Easy run 5 miles	•Low-impact cross-train	•Strength A + C •Easy run 5 miles
5	•Strength A + C •Easy run 4 miles	•Low-impact cross-train	•Strength B + C •Wild card (choose a workout from "Kick Your Own Butt" on page 155) or easy run 4 miles
6	•Strength B + C •Easy run 5 miles	•Low-impact cross-train	•Strength A + C •Easy run 6 miles
7	•Strength A + C •Easy run 6 miles	•Low-impact cross-train	•Strength B + C •Easy run 6 miles
8	•Strength B + C •Easy run 6 miles	•Low-impact cross-train	•Strength A + C •Wild card or easy run 6 miles
9	•Strength A + C •Easy run 5 miles	•Low-impact cross-train	•Strength B + C •Easy run 5 miles
10	•Strength B + C •Easy run 6 miles	•Low-impact cross-train	•Strength A + C •Wild card or easy run 7 miles
11	•Strength A + C •Easy run 6 miles	•Low-impact cross-train	•Strength B + C •Easy run 8 miles
12	•Strength B + C •Easy run 6 miles	•Low-impact cross-train	•Strength A + C •Easy run 6 miles
13	•Strength C •Easy run 6 miles	•Low-impact cross-train	•Strength C •Easy run 8 miles
14	•Strength C •Easy run 6 miles	•Low-impact cross-train	•Strength C •Easy run 8 miles
15	•Strength C •Easy run 4 miles	•Low-impact cross-train	•Strength C •Easy run 6 miles
16	•Rest	•Low-impact cross-train	•Easy run 4 miles

Thursday	Friday	Saturday	Sunday	Total
•Easy run 3 miles	•Strength A + C •Cross-train or rest	•Long run 6 miles	•Rest	16 miles
•Easy run 4 miles	•Strength B + C •Cross-train or rest	•Long run 8 miles	•Rest	20 miles
•Easy run 5 miles	•Strength A + C •Cross-train or rest	•Long run 10 miles	•Rest	24 miles
•Easy run 5 miles	•Strength B + C •Cross-train or rest	•Long run 12 miles	•Rest	27 miles
•Easy run 4 miles	•Strength A + C •Cross-train or rest	•Long run 10 miles	•Rest	22 miles˙
•Easy run 5 miles	•Strength B + C •Cross-train or rest	•Long run 14 miles	•Rest	30 miles
•Easy run 6 miles	•Strength A + C •Cross-train or rest	•Long run 15 miles	•Rest	33 miles
•Easy run 6 miles	•Cross-train or rest	•Long run 16 miles	•Rest	34 miles˙
•Easy run 5 miles	•Cross-train or rest	•Long run 11 miles	•Rest	26 miles
•Easy run 6 miles	•Cross-train or rest	•Long run 17 miles	•Rest	36 miles˙
•Easy run 6 miles	•Cross-train or rest	•Long run 18 miles	•Rest	38 miles
•Easy run 6 miles	•Cross-train or rest	•Long run 14 miles	•Rest	32 miles
•Easy run 6 miles	•Cross-train or rest	•Long run 20 miles	•Rest	40 miles
•Easy run 5 miles	•Cross-train or rest	•Long run 13 miles	•Rest	32 miles
•Easy run 4 miles	•Cross-train or rest	•Long run 8 miles	•Rest	22 miles
•Rest	•Easy run 2 miles	•Rest (this could also be race day)	•26.2 RACE DAY!	32.2 miles

˙ If you chose a wild-card workout this week you may have a different mileage total.

Intermediate In-Season Training Plan

Week	Monday	Tuesday	Wednesday
1	•Strength A + C •Easy run 3 miles	•Hilly run 4 miles	•Strength B + C
2	•Strength B + C •Easy run 3 miles	•Intermediate In-Season Fartlek (see page 164)	•Strength A + C
3	•Strength A + C •Easy run 4 miles	•Intermediate In-Season Track Ladder (see page 158)	•Strength B + C
4	•Strength B + C •Easy run 3 miles	**4 x 800** •Start with a 1-mile warm-up •Run each 800 at 30 seconds faster than your marathon race pace, with a 90-second walking recovery in between each 800 •End with a 1-mile cooldown	•Strength A + C •Easy run 3 miles
5	•Strength A + C •Easy run 4 miles	•Wild card (choose a workout from "Kick Your Own Butt" on page 155) or run 4 miles	•Strength B + C •Easy run 2 miles
6	•Strength B + C •Run 5 miles (2 miles at an easy pace, then 2 miles at marathon pace, then 1 mile at an easy pace)	**12 X 400** •Start with a 1-mile warm-up •Run each 400 at 10K pace •End with a 1-mile cooldown	•Strength A + C •Easy run 4 miles
7	•Strength A + C •Easy run 4 miles	•6 miles (run mile one at easy pace, run miles 2–5 at tempo pace, run mile six at easy pace)	•Strength B + C •Easy run 2 miles
8	•Strength B + C •Easy run 6 miles	•Wild card or easy run 6 miles	•Strength A + C •Easy run 4 miles
9	•Strength A + C •Easy run 5 miles	•5 miles (2 miles at an easy pace, then 2 miles at marathon pace, then 1 mile at an easy pace)	•Strength B + C •Easy run 5 miles
10	•Strength B + C •Easy run 4 miles	•Intermediate In-Season 5 x 1,000 (see page 160)	•Strength A + C •Easy run 6 miles
11	•Strength A + C •Easy run 7 miles	•Wild card or easy run 7 miles	•Strength B + C •Easy run 4 miles

Thursday	Friday	Saturday	Sunday	Total
·Cross-train or rest	·Strength A + C ·3 easy miles	·Long run 8 miles	·Rest	18 miles
·Cross-train or rest	·Strength B + C ·Easy run 3 miles	·Long run 10 miles	·Rest	20 miles
·Cross-train or rest	·Strength A + C ·Easy run 2 miles	·Long run 13 miles	·Rest	24 miles
·Cross-train or rest	·Strength B + C ·Easy run 2 miles	·Long run 13 miles	·Rest	25 miles
·Cross-train or rest	·Strength A + C ·Easy run 4 miles	·Long run 10 miles	·Rest	24 miles*
·Cross-train or rest	·Strength B + C ·Easy run 3 miles	·Long run 14 miles	·Rest	31 miles
·Easy run 4 miles	·Strength A + C ·Cross-train or rest	·Long run 16 miles	·Rest	32 miles
·Easy run 6 miles	·Cross-train or rest	·Run a half-marathon! (I suggest adding a 2-mile warm-up and 1-mile cooldown)	·Rest	35.1 miles*
·Cross-train or rest	·Easy run 5 miles	·Long run 11 miles	·Rest	26 miles
·Cross-train or rest	·Easy run 3 miles	·Long run 18 miles	·Rest	39 miles
·Cross-train or rest	·Easy run 2 miles	·Long run 18 miles	·Rest	38 miles*

* If you chose a wild-card workout this week you may have a different mileage total.

Week	Monday	Tuesday	Wednesday
12	•Strength B + C •Easy run 3 miles	**Mile Repeats** •Run 2 miles at an easy pace to warm up •Run 1 mile starting at half-marathon pace and gradually getting faster (aim to hit 5K pace in the last quarter mile) •Repeat this for 3 more miles •Run 1 easy mile to cool down	•Strength A + C •Easy run 3 miles
13	•Strength C •Easy run 6 miles	•Intermediate In-Season Hill Pusher (see page 162)	•Strength C •Easy run 5 miles
14	•Strength C •Easy run 6 miles	•Wild card or easy run 5 miles	•Strength C •Easy run 4 miles
15	•Strength C •Easy run 4 miles	**4 x 800** •Start with a 1-mile warm-up •Run each 800 at half-marathon pace •End with a 1-mile cooldown	•Strength C •Easy run 4 miles
16	•Rest	**200/400 Shakeout** •Start with a half-mile warm-up •Run 2 x 200 at marathon pace; jog back to the start after each repetition •Run 1 x 400 at marathon pace; jog back to the start •Run 2 x 200 at marathon pace; jog back to the start after each repetition •End with a half-mile cooldown	•Easy run 2 miles

Thursday	Friday	Saturday	Sunday	Total
•Cross-train or rest	•Hilly run 6 miles	•Long run 14 miles	•Rest	33 miles
•Cross-train or rest	•Easy run 4 miles	•Long run 20 miles	•Rest	43 miles
•Cross-train or rest	•Easy run 4 miles	•Long run 13 miles	•Rest	32 miles*
•Cross-train or rest	•Easy run 2 miles	•Long run 8 miles	•Rest	22 miles
•Rest	•Easy run 2 miles	•Rest (this could also be race day)	•26.2 RACE DAY!	32.2 miles

* If you chose a wild-card workout this week you may have a different mileage total.

Advanced In-Season Training Plan

Week	Monday	Tuesday	Wednesday
1	•Strength A + C •Easy run 4 miles	**12 x 400** •Start with a 1-mile warm-up •Run each 400 at 10K pace, with a 90-second jogging rest between each 400 •End with a 1-mile cooldown	•Strength B + C •Easy run 4 miles
2	•Strength B + C •Easy run 6 miles	•Hilly run 5 miles (accelerate on both uphills and downhills)	•Strength A + C •Easy run 4 miles
3	•Strength A + C •Easy run 8 miles	•Wild card (choose a workout from "Kick Your Own Butt" on page 155) or easy run 5 miles	•Strength B + C •Easy run 5 miles
4	•Strength B + C •Easy run 8 miles	•Advanced In-Season Fartlek (see page 164)	•Strength A + C •Easy run 5 miles
5	•Strength A + C •Easy run 8 miles	**5 tempo miles** •Start with a 2-mile warm-up •Run 5 miles at tempo pace •End with a 1-mile cooldown	•Strength B + C •Easy run 4 miles
6	•Strength B + C •Easy run 8 miles	**24 x 200** •Start with a 2-mile warm-up •Run each 200 at 10K pace, with a 200-meter jogging recovery between each 200 •End with a 1-mile cooldown	•Strength A + C •Easy run 8 miles
7	•Strength A + C •Easy run 8 miles	**3 X 2 miles at half-marathon pace** •Start with a 1-mile warm-up •Run two miles at half-marathon pace •Jog for 1 minute •Repeat this sequence twice more •End with a 1-mile cooldown	•Strength B + C •Easy run 7 miles
8	•Strength B + C •Easy run 6 miles	•Advanced In-Season Track Ladder (see page 160)	•Strength A + C •Easy run 5 miles
9	•Strength A + C •Easy run 8 miles	•Advanced In-Season 5 x 1,000 (see page 160)	•Strength B + C •Easy run 8 miles

Thursday	Friday	Saturday	Sunday	Total
•Cross-train or rest	•Strength A + C •Easy run 6 miles	•Long run 10 miles at easy pace	•Rest	29 miles
•Cross-train or rest	•Strength B + C •Hilly run 7 miles	•Long run 10 miles	•Rest	32 miles
•Cross-train or rest	•Strength A + C •Hilly run 8 miles	•Long run 12 miles	•Rest	38 miles*
•Cross-train or rest	•Strength B + C •Easy run 8 miles	•Long run 12 miles	•Rest	38 – 45 miles
•Cross-train or rest	•Strength A + C •Hilly run 7 miles	•Long run 12 miles	•Rest	39 miles
•Cross-train or rest	•Strength B + C •Easy run 7 miles	•Long run 14 miles	•Rest	46 miles
•Cross-train or rest	•Strength A + C •Hilly run 8 miles	**Long run: fartlek 15 miles** •Run the first 8 miles relaxed •Run fartleks for the next 5 miles, alternating between 30 seconds at faster than marathon pace, thirty seconds at marathon pace, and thirty seconds at slower than marathon pace •Finish with a 2-mile cooldown	•Rest	46 miles
•Cross-train or rest	•Easy run 5 miles	•Run a half-marathon! (I suggest adding a 2-mile warm-up and 1-mile cooldown)	•Rest	39.1 miles
•Cross-train or rest	•Hilly run 7 miles	•Long run 16 miles	•Rest	44 miles

* If you chose a wild-card workout this week you may have a different mileage total.

Week	Monday	Tuesday	Wednesday
10	•Strength B + C •Easy run 8 miles	•Wild card or easy run 6 miles	•Strength A + C •Easy run 8 miles
11	•Strength A + C •Easy run 8 miles	•Advanced In-Season Michigan (see page 166)	•Strength B + C •Easy run 7 miles
12	•Strength B + C •Easy run 8 miles	**8 X 800 hills** •Run a 1-mile warm-up •Run the following 8 times: uphill 400 and downhill 400 at 10K pace •Walk for 2 minutes to recover between each repeat •Run a 1-mile cooldown	•Strength A + C •Easy run 7 miles
13	•Strength C •Easy run 8 miles	**5 x 1 mile** •Run a 3-mile warm-up •Complete 5 1-mile repeats at half-marathon pace •Rest for 2 minutes between each repeat •Finish with a 2-mile cooldown	•Strength C •Easy run 8 miles
14	•Strength C •Easy run 8 miles	•Wild card or easy run 5 miles	•Strength C •Easy run 8 miles
15	•Strength C •Easy run 5 miles	**6 x 800** •Run a 1.5-mile warm-up •Run each 800 at half marathon pace •Jog a 400 between each repeat •Finish with a 1-mile cooldown	•Easy run 4 miles
16	•Easy run 4 miles	**2 x 1 mile** •Run a 1-mile warm-up •Run 1 mile at marathon pace •Rest 90 seconds •Run 1 mile at marathon pace •Run a 1-mile cooldown	•Easy run 4 miles

As you look at your plan, think about how much stronger you are going to be by race day. You've made it through the hardest part already. Now it's time to get you in race shape! This is where the fun is and the magic happens. Let's go!

Thursday	Friday	Saturday	Sunday	Total
•Cross-train or rest	•Easy run 5 miles	•Long run 17 miles (7 miles at an easy pace, then 5 miles at marathon pace, then 5 miles at an easy pace)	•Rest	44 miles*
•Cross-train or rest	•Easy run 5 miles	•Long run 18 miles	•Rest	51 miles
•Cross-train or rest	•Easy run 6 miles	•Long run 15 miles •Run 7 easy miles •Then run 7 miles at marathon pace •Finish with 1 easy mile	•Rest	42 miles
•Cross-train or rest	•Easy run 8 miles	•Long run 20 miles	•Rest	54 miles
•Cross-train or rest	•Easy run 7 miles	•18 miles (12–16 of them at marathon pace)	•Rest	46 miles*
•Rest	•Easy run 5 miles	•Long run 10 miles	•Rest	30.75 miles
•Rest	•Easy run 3 miles	•Rest (this could also be race day)	•26.2 RACE DAY!	41.2 miles

* If you chose a wild-card workout this week you may have a different mileage total.

GET STRONG(ER)!

You've made it through your base training months and you're ready to embark on a new journey. I know you're anxious to get out there and run forever, get faster, and crush high-mileage weeks. But don't drop the dumbbells yet. We need to seamlessly integrate a new strength routine into your training. Maybe you found the workouts easy while you were building your base. That's rad.

If that sounds like you, then we simply need to maintain your gains during the next four months of training. But I hear you—adding an additional thirty minutes of exercise on top of the enormous time spent on the road, paired with your already hectic weekly schedule of work and life, sounds like a real slog. But come on, stay with me. Dr. Kaci Brandt, a physical therapist and running coach with a PhD in physical therapy, tells it like it is: "What you're putting yourself through is a whole-body experience. And running is just a fourth of your marathon training plan. If you're only running, you are neglecting other vital aspects that support your muscles and brain as you pound away."

Kaci is part of a collective of female coaches called Lift Run Perform. She's an eight-time marathoner, a triathlete, and a Half Ironman finisher. She's also very competitive, which stems from her time as a figure skater on the Canadian national team. She knows how to train, race, compete, and rehab injuries. The number one mistake Kaci says marathoning women make is deprioritizing strength training. Inevitably, these runners end up in her office. The thing is, she understands. It happened to her: While training for her second full marathon (with no strength added), she experienced a terrible pain in her foot that she thought might be a tear. It was small, but it left her in a boot for six weeks. She didn't sit on the couch, though. Instead, she kept her cardio up by cycling and added in a few body-weight and free-weight exercises. She healed a few weeks before the marathon, and while she knew it wouldn't be her best time, her fitness was good enough that she decided to go for it. When she got to the finish, she was surprised by how fresh her legs were. "I felt so strong," she says. "I thought about how great I might feel by keeping up the strength program while running the proper number of miles."

THE RIGHT FORMULA

One thing Kaci harps on is the importance of a running-specific strength plan. "Sometimes the women I coach tell me that they go to a HIIT class or do a generic circuit-training session. But that's not hitting the key muscle groups. Plus, it could put unnecessary strain on your body."

Right. Two million burpees aren't going to help you perform better. We're already gaining cardiovascular endurance through running, and we don't need to add much more jumping and pounding during heavy-mileage weeks. So let's get focused. First we need to discuss the posterior chain—the muscles in your back body.

"The whole back body is your powerhouse," Kaci says. Translation: glutes and hamstrings. Many of us are quad dominant, so engaging our hamstrings and getting them balanced will not only add power but also protect against muscle strain.

Core strength fits into this equation too. No, not six-pack abs. That might be a nice side effect, but it's never the goal. We need our core muscles to stabilize our lower extremities and keep our hips, knees, and ankles aligned.

Finally, female runners have notoriously tight, and sometimes weak, hips. Opening and strengthening the hip flexors is essential. If you think about how many times we use our hips to lift our knees, it's no wonder they feel used and abused. Pair that with the annoying fact that most of us are required to sit all day, and you have a recipe for tightness. Kaci says tightness is the precursor to pain.

Our plan targets these areas and maintains the strength you created during the base months. You'll notice there are a lot of moves that require balance, which Kaci added to ensure we're really stabilizing our core and making both sides of our body balanced. The best practice is to implement the program in phases, meaning the load and frequency should be adjusted depending on what segment of training you're in.

Weeks 1–7: Low-to-moderate-mileage weeks. Complete a strength circuit three times per week (Monday, Wednesday, Friday), alternating between Strength A and Strength B. The Strength C circuit is a maintenance strength program. Please do the moves from Strength C anytime you do Strength A or Strength B.

Weeks 8–12: High-mileage weeks. Complete the strength circuits two times per week, alternating between Strength A and Strength B, on Mondays and Wednesdays. Do the moves in Strength C both days.

Weeks 13–16: Taper: Back off strength programming. Do the moves from Strength C two times per week, on Mondays and Wednesdays. In the week leading up to the race, don't worry about strength training.

STRENGTH A

Complete three sets of this circuit in the order below:

Body-Weight Good Mornings

10 repetitions

A great move for your deep core and back, this exercise will feel as good as it sounds. Stand with your feet shoulder width apart. Place your hands behind your head, elbows out wide, like you're about to get frisked. Stand tall, brace your core, and expand your shoulder blades. Inhale and bend forward. You want to maintain a flat back and hinge from your hips. Keep a slight bend in your knees. Return to standing.

Body-Weight Squats

10 repetitions

Start standing with your feet about shoulder width apart. Extend your hands straight out in front of you. Then bend your knees and push your hips and butt back, almost as though you're lowering yourself into an imaginary chair. Keep your chest lifted, your back straight, and your heels on the ground. Make sure your knees stay directly over your ankles—you don't want your knees to go too far forward. Aim to get your knees to a ninety-degree angle. Then push through your heels to stand back up.

Diagonal Lunges

10 repetitions on each leg, alternating

Stand tall with your feet hip distance apart and your hands on your hips. In a forward lunge, you'd step in front of you. In this variation, imagine you're facing toward twelve o'clock. Step your right foot across toward the ten o'clock position and lower into a lunge. Step back to the center. Step your left foot toward the two o'clock position and lower into a lunge. Your legs should be parallel to each other. Continue to alternate legs. (Both legs should complete ten repetitions.)

Single-Leg Dead Lifts

10 repetitions on each leg

Put your balance, strength, and focus to the test. From an athletic stance, bend forward (making sure to hinge from your hips) and lift your left leg behind you so you're balancing on your right leg. Keep your right knee slightly bent to load your glutes and hamstrings. Reach down and touch your left hand toward the ground. Return to standing and, without letting your left foot touch the floor, bend your left knee and draw it up toward your chest. Then allow your left knee to come back down (but don't let your left foot touch the ground!) and bend forward again, hinging from your hips, lifting your left leg behind you so you are balancing on your right leg. Finally, come back to standing on both legs. Switch so that you're balancing on your left leg, and repeat.

Plank Rows

10 repetitions on each arm

Big bang for your buck with this move, which will help prevent core rotation while you run. Get into high plank position with a dumbbell in each hand. Lift your right dumbbell up like you're elbowing someone behind you. Your hand should come to the right side of your rib cage and your elbow should be pointing up to the sky. Lower the dumbbell back to the ground. Important: If you feel your hips swaying to the side, ditch the weights. Maintaining proper alignment is the goal here. Repeat the movement on the left side.

Push-ups

10 repetitions

You know how to do a push-up. Go for it!

Low Plank

Hold for 30 seconds, rest for 30 seconds,
then hold for another 30 seconds.

Position yourself like you're about to do a push-up, but instead of placing your hands on the floor, place your forearms on the floor. Your elbows should be below your shoulders. You can place your palms flat on the ground or clasp your hands together. Your feet should be apart, in line with your shoulders. Engage your core, squeezing the muscles in your abs and glutes so that they stabilize your whole body. Ground the toes into the floor.

Low Side Plank

Hold for 30 seconds on the right side, rest for 30 seconds,
then switch sides and hold for 30 seconds on the left side.
Repeat this sequence one more time before moving on.

For this plank variation, start on your side, with your feet together and your right elbow directly below your shoulder. Raise your hips so that your body is in a straight line from head to feet. Place your left hand on your hip. Your right forearm and feet should be the only parts of your body touching the ground. Hold this position. You should feel this in your obliques, which are the muscles on the sides of your abs. These do wonders for helping you maintain stability in your core while running.

STRENGTH B

These are supersets, meaning you will perform repetitions of one exercise immediately following another exercise to make up a full set. These particular supersets are designed to work opposing muscle groups, which gives you the benefit of getting more work done with less rest without exhausting yourself.

Instructions:

- Do twelve repetitions of the first exercise in superset 1 (lateral squat).
- Then immediately do twelve repetitions of the second move in superset 1 (triceps dip).
- Take a ten-second rest.
- Move on to superset 2.
- Do twelve repetitions of each exercise in superset 2 (with no rest between the two exercises), then take a ten-second rest.
- Do twelve repetitions of each exercise in superset 3 (with no rest between the two exercises), then take a ten-second rest.
- Do twelve repetitions of each exercise in superset 4 (with no rest between the two exercises), then take a ten-second rest.
- When you have completed all four supersets, take a one-minute rest.
- Repeat this cycle four times.
- At the end of the fourth cycle, complete the Core Bonus.

Superset 1

Lateral Squat: This is a yummy move that should torch your hip flexors. Stand with your feet shoulder width apart. Place your hands on your hips or behind your head. Step out to the right and shift your body weight over to your right leg. Keeping your chest high, squat so that your right knee makes a ninety-degree angle. Your left leg will be straight. Sink your butt low.

Triceps Dip: Sit on the edge of a secured bench or stable chair. Gripping the edge of the bench or chair, position your hands shoulder width apart, on either side of your hips. Slide your butt off the front of the chair or bench with your legs extended out in front of you. Straighten your arms, keeping a little bend in your elbows. At this point, you should feel tension on your triceps—not your elbow joints. Slowly bend your elbows to lower your body toward the floor until your elbows are (ideally) at about a ninety-degree angle. Be sure to keep your back close to the bench. Once you reach the bottom, push yourself back up to the start position and repeat.

Superset 2

Reverse Lunge: Starting from an athletic stance, step your left foot behind you and keep your left heel lifted. Lower your hips so that your right thigh is parallel to the floor. Check that your right knee is in line with your ankle. Do one set on the same leg, then switch legs the next time around.

Hammer Curl: While in a standing position, hold a set of dumbbells by your sides with your knuckles facing out (your palms should face inward). Your elbows should be tucked in to your sides. Curl both forearms up while keeping your upper arms stationary. You want to bring the weights up to shoulder level, squeezing your biceps. Lower your arms down slowly. Repeat. If you find yourself using your hips to raise the dumbbells, grab a lower weight.

Superset 3

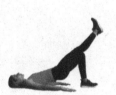

Single-Leg Bridge-Ups: Start by lying on your back with your left knee bent and your right leg straight. Squeeze your glutes and core to raise your hips and your right leg up into the air, keeping your right leg in line with your torso. Repeat all the reps with your left leg bent, then switch to the right on your next set.

Lying Lateral Leg Raise: Get down on the ground. Lie on your left side with the whole left side of your body touching the floor. Place your left arm straight on the floor under your head, or bend your elbow and use your left hand to support your head. Your body should be in a straight line, with your right leg stacked on top of your left. Lift your right leg into the air, then lower it back down to meet your left leg. Repeat all your reps on the right leg, then switch to your left on the next set.

Superset 4

Inchworms: Start by standing with your feet hip distance apart, then bend forward at your hips into a forward fold. Place your palms down on the ground, then walk your hands (in a million tiny steps, like you're an adorable, tiny worm) forward into high plank. Your hands should be under your shoulders and your feet still hip distance apart. Then walk your feet to meet your hands so that you're back in a forward fold. That's one. Stand up and repeat.

Fire Hydrants: Start in tabletop position, which means hands and knees on the floor, shoulder and hip-width distance apart, so that your back looks like a table. Engage your core and lift your leg to forty-five degrees without moving the rest of your body—like a male dog peeing on a fire hydrant. Get it? Again, do all reps on one leg, then switch to the other.

Core Bonus

High Plank

*Hold for 30 seconds, rest for 30 seconds,
then hold for 30 seconds.*

The high plank looks like the starting position for a push-up. Your palms should be on the floor and arms underneath you and in line with your shoulders. Your feet, knees, and quadriceps should be shoulder width apart and lifted off the ground. Maintain a neutral spine, meaning do not allow your butt to peak into the air or your hips to sag down toward the ground. Engage your core muscles (abs, back, and butt) to keep your body stable.

High Side Plank

Hold for 30 seconds on the right side,
rest for 30 seconds, then hold for 30 seconds
on the left side. Repeat this sequence one more time.

For this side-plank variation, start on your side, with your feet together and your right arm extended straight, palm on the ground. Raise your hips so that your body is in a straight line from head to feet. Place your left hand on your hip. Your right palm and feet should be the only parts of your body touching the ground. You should feel this in your obliques, which are the muscles on the sides of your abs. These do wonders for helping you maintain stability in your core while running.

High Reverse Plank

Hold for 30 seconds, rest for 30 seconds,
then hold for 30 seconds

Sit on the floor with your legs extended in front of you. Place your palms, with fingers spread wide, on the floor slightly behind and outside your hips. Press into your palms and lift your hips and torso toward the ceiling. Point your toes. Keep your arms and legs straight. Your body should form a straight line from your head to your heels. Squeeze your core and try to pull your belly button back toward your spine. If your hips begin to sag or drop, lower yourself back to the floor.

STRENGTH C

These moves are meant to maintain your strength, encourage core engagement, and keep the smaller muscle groups you use in running active and healthy. As I mentioned earlier, I recommend doing these almost every other day. They will not take more than ten minutes. Just make it a habit. I promise the results are worth it. Let's go!

Complete three sets of the following exercises:

10 Clamshells

Lie on your side with your hips and shoulders in a straight line, head resting on your bottom arm. Bring your knees toward your chest so that your thighs are at a ninety-degree angle to your body. Place your top hand on the floor in front of your chest for extra stability. Keeping your toes together, lift your top knee toward the ceiling. Your legs should look like a clam opening. Bring your knees together to the start position. Do five repetitions on one side, then five on the other side.

10 Single-Leg Bridge-Ups

Start by lying on your back with your left knee bent and right leg straight. Squeeze your glutes and core to raise your hips and your right leg up into the air. Hold for a count of two. Lower back down and repeat nine more times on the same leg. Switch sides and repeat.

20 Bird Dogs

From tabletop position, extend your right arm forward and left leg behind you (but don't put it up too high! keep it in line with the rest of you). Keep your head in line with your body, with your gaze down and your neck long. Inhale and hold for a beat. Lower and switch sides. Squeeze your abs and glutes when your limbs are extended. If you feel it too much in your lower back, you are likely lifting your leg too high.

10 Dead Bugs

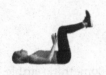

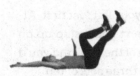

Lie flat on your back with your arms held out in front of you, pointing toward the ceiling. Then bring your legs up so your knees are bent at ninety-degree angles. This is your starting position. Make sure your back is as flat against the floor as possible. There shouldn't be a space between your lower spine and the ground. Slowly lower and straighten your right arm and left leg at the same time, exhaling as you go. Keep going until your right arm and left leg are just above the floor, being careful not to raise your back off the ground. Hold for one to two seconds. Then slowly return to the starting position and repeat with the opposite limbs. If your core is properly engaged, you should feel this in your lower back.

OPTIONAL MOVES TO PREVENT PAIN

If you've felt any pain while running or noticed little twinges of discomfort, that could mean an injury is imminent. If you have the means, then see your dang doctor and make sure it's nothing serious.

The thing is, a lot of minor injuries can be remedied with proper strength-training programs and rehab exercises. Even better, some little stretches and minimal work can prevent pain from troubling you at all. So if you want to be on the safe side, add these moves to the strength circuits or do them while you're watching TV.

IT Bands

Side Stretch: Stand with your left foot crossed behind your right foot. With your left arm overhead, bend to the right side. Hold for thirty seconds, then switch to the other side. Repeat three times per side.

Knees

Box Step-Ups: Find a sturdy box, chair, or couch—something stable and elevated that can support your weight. Step your right foot on top of it. Putting weight on your right foot, launch yourself off the ground until you're standing. Touch your left foot to the top of the box, then step back down to the ground with your left foot first. Alternate feet every repetition. For example, next you'd step up on your left foot, your right foot would tap the top of the box, and you'd step down with your right foot first. Complete three sets of ten.

Lower Back

Cat-Cow: This move is so underrated, but it opens up your back and your shoulders. Start in tabletop position. Exhale and round your spine up to the ceiling. Drop your head and release your neck. Then inhale and arch your back. Extend your head to the ceiling and broaden through the collarbone. Complete three sets of ten.

Slump Stretch: Sit on a chair. Hunch your shoulders and drop your chin to your chest. Lift one knee up so that your foot hovers over the floor. Hold for five seconds. Then repeat with the other leg. Complete the stretch five times per leg.

Hamstrings

Lying Hamstring Stretch: Every runner should just get in the practice of doing this stretch. Lie on your back. Lift one leg into the air with the other leg straight out on the floor. If you're tight through your hamstrings, allow the leg in the air to bend at the knee. You should feel this stretch in the upper back part of your thigh. Hold for thirty seconds, then switch legs. Repeat three times on each side.

Sitting Hamstring Stretch: While seated on the floor, extend your right leg out and keep your left leg bent with your left foot tucked into your right inner thigh. Reach your arms and chest over your right leg, and try to grab your toes with your hands. You should feel this behind your right knee and in the back lower part of your right thigh. Hold for thirty seconds, then switch legs. Repeat three times on each side.

Calves

Ankle Alphabet Soup: Get into a comfortable seated position. This could be in a chair, on a couch, or on the floor. Lift your right foot slightly above the ground just enough that it has space to move without hitting the floor. Using your ankle, draw the letters of the alphabet in the air with your foot. Try going through all the letters two times. Repeat on the other side.

Feet

Big-Toe Hug: Start seated in a chair. Put your right ankle on top of your left thigh. Grab your right big toe and gently pull it toward you.

Hold for thirty seconds. Do this three times, then switch and do the same with the other foot.

Towel Stretch: Hold a bath towel lengthwise to make an exercise strap. Sit on the ground with your legs stretched out in front of you. Your legs should be shoulder width apart. Place the towel under the arches of both feet. Grab the ends of the towel with both hands and pull your feet toward you while simultaneously pointing your toes. Your legs should stay on the ground. Hold for thirty seconds and repeat three times.

Weight Your Arches: My personal favorite. Get on your hands and knees on the floor. Keep your heels pointing up and the balls of your feet and your toes on the floor. Slowly sit back toward your ankles. You should feel a really nice release in your arches. Hold until it starts to feel uncomfortable, then release.

EMPOWER YOUR VAGINA

There is one aspect of strength that is seldom talked about. If you feel like you urgently need to pee while you're running, you're not alone. So many women have pelvic-floor issues, especially all my amazing mamas out there. The urgency or leakage might be a slight incontinence problem or something more serious, like a prolapse. Definitely see your ob-gyn, and know that it's not something you need to keep quiet. It's not embarrassing, it's really common, and it's totally fixable. The thing is, if you just ignore it, the pelvic-floor muscles will weaken, which could lead to more serious issues later on. In addition to seeing a doc, you can incorporate Kegels into your workouts. But a lot of women do Kegels incorrectly and perform the move by lifting their butt instead of the pelvic floor.

Try this instead: Start in a standing position, leaning slightly forward at your hips. Your ribs should be over your core and your tailbone should untuck. Start taking deep inhales and exhales. On an exhale, lift your pelvic floor by imagining your vagina picking up a small object. Your ab muscles will contract as well. Inhale and relax. Drop the imaginary object. Try this three times. If that's easy, do ten repetitions.

When you're doing your plank work, do the breathing and pelvic lift. These moves are for slight dysfunction and maintenance. If your pelvic-floor issue is persistent and affecting your performance, there are physical therapists who specialize in rehabbing this injury.

OVERCOMING THE STRENGTH BLOCK

If you're having trouble incorporating strength exercises into your routine, we need to identify the issue and challenge that weakness. Let's get to the bottom of what's going on.

You Lack Confidence

When Coach Mary Johnson, the founder of Lift Run Perform, gave a lecture at a women-only running retreat, she asked the audience a simple question: "Who here knows how to do a squat?" Nobody raised their hand. Coach Mary holds both USATF and VDOT O2 coaching certifications and is a Functional Range Conditioning mobility specialist. In addition to knowing quite a bit about physiology, she is an incredible runner who started with a marathon PR of 3:44 (fast) and dropped it to 3:06 (wowza). Anyway, she knows what she's talking about. At this retreat, after no one raised their hand, Mary asked the women to stand up. Without offering any instructions, she asked them to squat.

"Everyone could do a squat!" she says. She was flabbergasted. How could women who were perfectly competent at this very important movement doubt themselves? "It comes down to confidence," says Mary. She believes that this same self-doubt often keeps females from going to the gym or doing circuits on their own.

What's the remedy?

Identify what you think you don't know. Ask yourself, Have I done this before? Have I seen this before? Does my body know what muscles to engage and how to master the right form? Learning the move visually before you attempt to do it can make you feel more capable. Ask a trainer, a friend, or an Instagram fitfluencer, or simply turn to YouTube. There's no shame in asking questions, but don't be afraid to trust yourself.

You're Allergic to the Gym

Let's acknowledge that the gym can be intimidating. If the thought of elbowing your way to the free weights through a pack of beefy dudes staring at themselves in the mirror makes you break out in a cold sweat, know that you're not alone. But remember these two things. First, you belong there just as much as they do. In fact, you're probably in better shape than most of them. You are a tough-as-nails marathoner and you just need a pair of dumbbells. Second, these dudes are probably far too busy ogling their own muscles to care what you're doing. You just need to get your workout in.

If it's more the cost or lack of convenience that's keeping you from the gym, that's fine. Most of the exercises runners need can be done without a single piece of equipment. You can use your living room, your garage, or the road you're running down to get your reps and sets in. The world is your gym!

You Don't Have Time

"If you think you don't have time to add a few beneficial exercises to your running routine, then you need to make your goal a 5K," says Mary. She isn't messing around. You want to run 26.2, so let's brainstorm ways to fit this in.

1. Complete the moves right before you run. The proposed strength plans in here shouldn't take more than twenty minutes every day.
2. Skip your easy miles one day per week and do the strength work instead. Yes, really.

3. Just keep trying. Don't think that because you missed a day, all is lost. Aim to make strength a priority, and if you get a few squats and push-ups in, awesome. If you do it all and make it through three weeks, then it will become a habit and part of your routine.

You Fear Your Body Will Change . . . in a Bad Way

Good grief, do I even have to say this? YOU WON'T GET BULKY. Not with these moves. In fact, you'll probably look amazing. Plus, if you have an extrinsic goal of losing fat, adding a few strength moves will change your body composition faster than cardio alone.

You're Bored

Now, I know that doing the same strength-training circuit week after week gets tedious. Every once in a while, you can spice things up and break loose from the drudgery of lunges and planks. I asked my favorite fitness blogger and ultrarunner, Crystal Seaver, how she makes sure her workouts are both functional and fun. She adds exercises that challenge the muscles you need in running and work your brain too. Crystal knows what she's talking about—she's a personal trainer and coach who works with individuals and small groups through Relentless Runners. She got into the strength game after injuring herself on a long trail run. She makes sure her programming is fun but also supports her running goals. Here's an exciting, runner-specific grind she came up with. Trade it in for Strength A or Strength B whenever you need a challenge! She often posts what she's doing in the gym on Instagram, so if you're a fan of complex, high-power stuff, she's the gal for you.

Crystal's Workout

Complete one cycle of the following:

10 Banded Lateral Walks

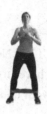

Place a resistance band around your shins, right above your ankles. Stand with your feet hip distance apart. Step your right foot out to the side, return to center, then step your left out. Continue moving back and forth. You should feel this work in your butt, core, and hips.

10 Low Squat Holds and Toe-Taps

Squat down. Keep your knees out and in line with your ankles. Hold! Then lift your right foot slightly and tap the floor. Switch sides.

20 Bear-Walking Crawls

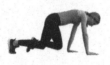

Start on all fours in tabletop position. Lift your knees so they hover an inch off the ground. You should immediately feel your abs light up. Lift your right hand and step it six inches in front of you. Simultaneously lift your left foot and step it six inches forward. Move your left hand forward to line up with your right and your right foot forward to line up with your left. Keep your core tight and stay low to the ground. You should look like a bear lumbering through the forest. After ten reps starting with your right hand and left foot, switch to lead with your left hand and right foot.

5 Pike Walks to Spider Taps

Start in high plank position, then walk your feet in so that your butt is high in the air. You should feel this in your core and shoulders. Now you're in pike position. From there, bring your right foot to where your right hand is planted, like Spider-Man. Return to pike position and then repeat on the other side.

20 Plank Shoulder Taps

In high plank position, keeping your pelvis and hips still, lift your right arm and tap your left shoulder. Return to high plank and repeat on the opposite side. If you start to sway, widen your legs. Pro tip: A wide-leg plank, sometimes called an RCL plank, is an amazing tool to work the deep core muscles and obliques. It maintains alignment and can improve posture in those with an anterior pelvic tilt, which many runners develop.

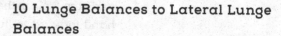

10 Lunge Balances to Lateral Lunge Balances

Lunge forward with your right leg. Bring your leg up and, without touching the floor, go into a side lunge position. Complete all the reps on one leg. Then switch. To modify, briefly touch your toe down while transitioning.

10 Lateral Walking Planks

While in a perfect high plank, walk your hands and feet to the right. Start by lifting the right hand and foot and "step" them over as far as you can (it does not have to be far). Rest for a beat in high plank. Take another "step" to the right, ending in high plank. Next, lift your left hand and foot and "step" to the left. Rest in high plank. Take another "step" to the left. That is one rep. This move can also be done on your knees with the same benefit.

10 Squat Cross Jumps

Drop into a squat position. While low, take your left hand and touch your right foot or shin. Jump up to standing. Drop down again and repeat on the alternate side. Use that core strength for balance!

10 Up-and-Down Planks

Start in high plank position. Then lower down onto your right forearm, then your left, into low plank. Rise back into high plank. That's one repetition.

10 Side Plank Tucks Each Side

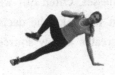

From high side plank position, extend your top arm over your head so your bicep is by your ear. Lift your top leg and squeeze your knee to your elbow, using your obliques. Repeat on the opposite side.

KICK YOUR OWN BUTT

You may have noticed that the in-season training plans include terms you might not recognize. Wild card? Fartlek?

Remember that time I told you to test yourself to find your weaknesses? Here is a handy section with loads of tough workouts that will make you say, "What weaknesses?" If you want to target any deficit, there is a workout in here for you. And if I know runners, then I know that sometimes you just want to do a workout that will cause your quads to ache the next day.

Years ago, when I decided to make a half-marathon my mission, I got the notion that I was finally a *serious* runner. Whatever that means. To confirm my seriousness, I read the classic running novel *Once a Runner*, which I highly recommend to any runner—regardless of the longest distance you've run. The chapter called "The Workout" has always stayed with me, and I think about it, even ten years later, every time I step onto a track.

In it, the protagonist, Cassidy, runs an insane 60 x 400. Ha! Remember how we tested ourselves by running six four hundreds? Could you imagine doing sixty of these? To ensure that I convey how insane this (fictional, do not try this IRL!) workout is, I must tell you that the true breakdown was 20 x 400 in sets of five, with a hundred-meter easy run between each four hundred and a four-hundred-meter jog between each set.

Look, I know that's an absurd workout. But I use it to inspire my will-power, determination, and excitement before my attempts at speedwork. I love the idea of aggressively pushing up against human limits, because when you brush up against your threshold, you often experience a break-through. That's why I believe in uncovering weaknesses. Often our weaknesses are just what we perceive as difficult. When we make the decision to home in on something that challenges us, it creates a new source of power.

All of us have breakthrough moments in running. No matter if you started two months or twenty years ago, you can recall a time when you set out to run something that seemed impossible and then crushed it. Maybe it was when you ran ten miles for the first time. Or perhaps you finally made it up the hill in your neighborhood without walking. First and foremost, it's important to recognize and identify those moments. Think about a run that made you feel completely unstoppable.

Write it down here:

_____

_____

I asked all the coaches and marathoners who contributed to this book if they could remember one of those workouts that made them feel like a metallic rainbow fish. Some people recalled just everyday training runs where they got into the zone. One runner said it was a pain-free run following an injury. Coach Ashlee Lawson was thrown out of a van on a running retreat and had to run up a mountain. Other coaches offered specific workouts that kicked their butts and that gave them true confidence in their running ability. These are the workouts they wanted to share. Some of these runs are advanced. Some are simply fun. Others are traditional gut busters that will give you a sense of power and long-lasting confidence.

The idea here is that by incorporating some of these super tough workouts into your repertoire, you broaden the possibility of experiencing your own breakthrough moment during this training cycle. Even if you don't feel some sort of otherworldly inspiration while running these, the very act of completing one of them should signal to you just how incredible you are. That's why I want you to choose a power word or phrase and repeat it to yourself while you do these runs. This will bookmark the feeling of awesomeness in your mind so you can later call upon it when you need it most. (Think: you need to crush a hill in the race, so you think of your power word and recall that time you defeated pain and triumphed over your toughest workout. You see what I'm saying?)

Power Word/Phrase Examples

Go	Free	Grit
Turn it on	Activate	Courage
Fire	Rock-solid	Crush it
Conquer	Let's do this	Focus
Heart	Burn	Forward
Up	In it	
Be light	Love	

Keep the phrase short, perhaps no longer than three syllables. Some people also think of a visual to go with the word. For example, I use *heart*, and when I need to recall my inner strength, my great breakthroughs, I will imagine a beating heart with light overflowing from its edges. Try it!

You know, aside from the confidence boost, these workouts help your running in real, physical ways. Many mix together various techniques to boost strength, aerobic capacity, anaerobic capacity, VO2 max, and speed endurance.

Track Ladder

A track ladder is such a great confidence booster because it shows you that you can run on tired, wobbly legs. It gives you all the physical benefits of interval work. And of course, if you don't have a track, find a nice, long stretch of road where you can mark distances. You will hate going "up" the ladder, but believe me, the glory of making it to the "top" of the ladder and riding the shorter distances back down will leave you smiling.

Classic Track Ladder

Start with a fifteen-minute warm-up run at a very slow pace and complete a dynamic warm-up.* Then complete the following intervals at a 5K pace. During the rest periods, try to maintain movement by either jogging or walking. Finish with a gentle ten-minute cooldown.

> 200 m → 0:30 recovery
> 400 m → 1:00 recovery
> 800 m → 1:30 recovery
> 1,200 m → 2:00 recovery
> 1,600 m → 4:00 recovery
> 1,200 m → 2:00 recovery
> 800 m → 1:30 recovery
> 400 m → 1:00 recovery
> 200 m → celebration

Intermediate In-Season Track Ladder

Start with a fifteen-minute warm-up run at a very slow pace and complete a dynamic warm-up. Then complete the following intervals at a 10K pace. During the rest periods, try to maintain movement by either jogging or walking. Finish with a gentle one-mile cooldown.

> 200 m → 0:30 recovery
> 400 m → 1:00 recovery
> 800 m → 1:30 recovery
> 1,200 m → 2:00 recovery
> 1,200 m → 2:00 recovery
> 800 m → 1:30 recovery
> 400 m → 1:00 recovery
> 200 m → celebration

---

* For a full dynamic warm-up, go back to chapter 4 on page 25.

Advanced In-Season Track Ladder

Start with a one-mile warm-up run at a very slow pace and complete a dynamic warm-up. Then complete the following intervals at a 10K pace. Try to maintain movement by either jogging or walking. However, during the five-minute break between sets, walk or stretch. Finish with a gentle one-mile cooldown.

400 m → 1:00 recovery
800 m → 1:30 recovery
1,200 m → 2:00 recovery
1,600 m → 3:00 recovery
1,200 m → 2:00 recovery
800 m → 1:30 recovery
400 m → 5:00 break
400 m → 1:00 recovery
800 m → 1:30 recovery
1,200 m → 2:00 recovery
1,600 m → 3:00 recovery
1,200 m → 2:00 recovery
800 m → 1:30 recovery
400 m → celebration

5 x 1,000

If you've been running for a hot minute, you might look at this workout and recognize it as a tool for 5K training. You're right! If you've ever completed a 5 x 1,000, then you also know that it's a beast. It helps spur aerobic endurance, improves leg turnover, and recruits fast- and slow-twitch muscles.

Classic 5 x 1,000

Run a 1-mile warm-up.
Run 1,000 meters at 5K pace.

Do a 400-meter active-recovery jog.

Repeat 4 more times.

Run a 1-mile cooldown.

Intermediate/Advanced In-Season 5 x 1,000

Run a 1-mile warm-up.

Run 1,000 meters at half-marathon pace.

Walk for 90 seconds between each interval.

Repeat 4 more times.

Rest for 4 minutes.

Run 5 more 1,000-meter intervals at half-marathon pace.

Run a 1-mile cooldown.

Race-Pace Long Run Ladder

If you're an experienced runner, adding a few miles at race pace to the longest runs of your week will be incorporated in your plan already. If you're newish to marathoning but still want to work on feeling out race-pace miles, try adding the following sequence into mile two of any run that is five miles or more. If you finish the sequence with miles to go, finish off the run at an easy pace. If your prescribed miles come before you get to the last sequence, end the run where you are (i.e., don't add miles to finish the ladder). If this happens, do make sure to cool down, even if it's just a five-minute walk. If you add visualization and the tool of a power word to this workout, you will be able to feel the pace you need to run on race day, which will increase the likelihood that you'll reach flow state.

2 minutes at race pace, 1 minute easy

4 minutes at race pace, 2 minutes easy

6 minutes at race pace, 3 minutes easy

6 minutes at race pace, 3 minutes easy

6 minutes at race pace, 3 minutes easy

4 minutes at race pace, 2 minutes easy

2 minutes at race pace, 1 minute easy

Hill Pusher

Classic Hill Pusher

For this workout, you want to find a six-mile route with a few hills of various sizes. Use the first mile as your warm-up, then prime your hips, butt, and quads with the dynamic warm-up. You want these muscle groups to be alive and awake to tackle hills. After warming up, you should have five miles left to run. For these five miles, you want to accelerate up every hill at tempo pace. Recover at the top with a light, slow jog, then quickly settle back into your easy pace. Even if you cannot reach tempo pace while going up every hill, still try to accelerate while keeping proper form. Cool down with a five-minute walk. This is an exhausting workout, and you may need to take a full day off the following day.

Intermediate In-Season Hill Pusher

When you encounter the Hill Pusher in the intermediate training plan, it is very similar to the Classic Hill Pusher—just longer and at a slightly slower pace.

Complete a one-mile warm-up and a dynamic warm-up. Start at easy pace but focus on accelerating up the hills at half-marathon pace. Recover at the top with a light, slow jog, then quickly settle back into your easy pace. Complete six miles. Finish with a one-mile cooldown.

Happy Hill Sprints

Hill sprints will bring out the fighter in you. If you have a good running friend, make them do it with you. The company makes the work much more fun and keeps you accountable. Find a hill with a 10 percent grade. Honestly, if you look at a hill and say, "Oh, that's steep," then that will probably work for what we're trying to accomplish, which is building both power and speed. The form for hill sprints doesn't change from what you learned during the hill test (see page 82), but your cadence will quicken. These are sprints, after all. When you're running uphill, drive your knees forward toward your chest and land on the balls of your feet. Lean slightly forward and pump your arms. Try to keep your shoulders away from your ears, stay relaxed, and keep your core tight. Go all out. Your breath will be ragged—just make sure you do actually breathe!

> Run a 1-mile warm-up and complete a dynamic warm-up.
> Start at the bottom of your hill and accelerate up for 12 to 15 seconds.
> Float back to the bottom.
> Rest for no less than 20 seconds and no more than 90 seconds.
> Repeat 9 more times (for a total of 10).
> Run a 1-mile cooldown.

If you are able to convince a friend to do the work with you, making it a relay and tagging each other at the bottom will help the reps go by faster, will ensure no one is resting for too long, and might help you keep track of how many sprints you have to go.

Fartlek

Fartlek, a Swedish word, means "speed play." The point of fartlek runs is that they are constantly varied, to prevent both psychological and physiological boredom. So in a sense, it is playful and really fun. It's most common to vary the speed, but you can also vary the terrain. So what does *vary* mean? How fast should you go and for how long? Below are a few variations.

Classic Five-Mile Fartlek

For this exercise, forget about your pace calculator and think about your paces more generally as four different categories: easy, medium, medium-hard, and hard. After one easy mile and a dynamic warm-up, begin to run at a medium pace (think of this as your most comfortable pace—not slow, not fast). After you find your groove, choose a physical object in the distance, for example, a tree. Slow down and run to your object at a slow, easy pace. Once you reach it, pick something new—maybe a mailbox—and from the tree to the mailbox, run at a medium-hard pace (slightly faster than might be comfortable). Once you make it to the mailbox, relax into your medium pace, then pick a new destination where you will ramp up to a fast, hard pace. Continue along, shifting from different paces at different times. Jump from easy to hard, hard to medium-hard, then go easy, then medium, then easy again. If that sounds confusing, good. But if it sounds like straight chaos, just alternate easy, medium, and hard until you get the hang of this whole fartlek thing. The general idea is to run the next three miles at somewhat random paces, settling into a normal cadence for a minute and then playing with your speed. If picking objects sounds annoying, you can accomplish the same effect by counting down seconds or even minutes (see plans below). After three miles of roller-coaster running, slow it down and finish with a steady cooldown mile.

Intermediate In-Season Fartlek

Complete a one-mile warm-up. The next two miles will be timed fartlek, following the pattern below.

> 90 seconds easy
> 60 seconds medium-hard
> Alternate between these two speeds until you hit a total of 3 miles.
> Finish with a 1-mile cooldown.

Advanced In-Season Fartlek

Complete a one-mile warm-up. Then run the following pattern:

> 60 seconds easy
> 60 seconds medium

60 seconds hard
60 seconds easy
60 seconds medium
60 seconds hard
60 seconds easy
60 seconds medium
60 seconds hard
60 seconds easy
60 seconds medium
60 seconds hard
60 seconds easy
60 seconds medium
Complete a 1-mile cooldown.

The Michigan

Coach Ellen London, who hails from Boston and is a coach for Heartbreak Hill Running Company's Heartbreaker Run Club, couldn't say the words fast enough when I asked for the hardest workout she's ever done. The Michigan, she told me, is a notorious workout that combines various training methods into one ungodly session. You'll switch paces and terrains and simulate race-day segments. It was originally used among college track athletes but has since made its way into the routines of pedestrian runners. Ellen's an old pro at the Michigan now and advises that marathoners attempt it five or six weeks away from race day. "If you can run it," she says, "you can basically get through anything."

Warm up.
Run 1 mile around a track at 10K pace.
Slow down for 2 to 3 minutes, using this time to leave the track and
    slowly run to a sidewalk, trail, dirt road, anywhere off track where
    you can run.
Run a mile somewhere off track at tempo pace.

Return to the track in a slow jog (you're aiming to slow jog for approximately 1 mile).

Back on the track, run 1,200 meters at 10K pace.

Slow jog away from the track, again taking no more than 3 minutes.

Repeat the same off-track mile at tempo pace.

Jog back to the track (the 1 mile back).

Back on the track, run 800 meters at 10K pace.

Jog away from the track, taking no more than 4 minutes.

Repeat the same off-track mile at tempo pace.

Jog back to the track (the 1 mile back).

Back at the track, run 400 meters as if it were the last quarter mile
  of your goal race.

Peel yourself off the finish line and revel in your own brilliance.

Advanced In-Season Michigan

Follow the instructions for the Michigan above, but start with a three-mile
warm-up and end with a two-mile cooldown.

Nearly Never-Ending Tabata

The idea for Tabata training started with speed skaters. Dr. Izumi Tabata, a
professor at the Graduate School of Sport and Health Science at Ritsumeikan University in Japan, set out to study the most efficient way to improve
VO2 max. He prescribed a short burst of high-intensity exercise, followed
by even shorter rests. The format is twenty seconds of all-out work and ten
seconds of rest. You perform the sequence eight times for a total of four
minutes. You might think it sounds easy, but those small time increments
are deceiving. If you're not drenched in sweat by the end of a Tabata session,
then you're probably not doing it right. Here's how to adapt it for distance
running.

Run an easy warm-up mile and complete your dynamic warm-up.

Next, run hard for 20 seconds, followed by a 10-second jog.

Do that 7 more times (8 repetitions is considered 1 Tabata).

Run an easy mile.

Repeat the Tabata.

Run an easy half mile.

Repeat the Tabata.

Run an easy quarter mile.

Repeat the Tabata.

Cool down for 5 minutes.

Two-Mile Torture

When my running BFF, Hannah McGoldrick, was about five weeks away from running the Toronto Marathon, she looked at her plan and saw this beast of a workout. It demands 10K pace, which should be quicker than your marathon pace and will work your speed-endurance capabilities hard. Hannah went out and did the work. "The fact that I accomplished it and hit my paces made me think to myself, 'Shoot, I am ready for this marathon.'" Not only was she ready, but she ended up running a thirteen-minute PR. Maybe you're tough enough to have a breakthrough moment during this workout too.

Run a 1.5-mile easy warm-up

Run 2 miles at 10K pace.

Take a 60-second active recovery.

Run 2 more miles at 10K pace.

Take a 60-second active recovery.

Run 2 more miles at 10K pace.

Complete a 1.5-mile cooldown.

Power Hour

This is a hodgepodge of exercises designed to replicate a HIIT routine. While this might not be the most effective way to train for a marathon, it is a mood booster.

Warm-up
15 push-ups
1 mile at 10K pace
30-second rest
20 burpees
1 mile at 10K pace
30-second rest
10 push-ups
1 mile at 10K pace
30-second rest
15 burpees
1 mile at 5K pace
30-second rest
5 push-ups
800 meters at 5K pace
30-second rest
10 burpees
800 meters at 5K pace
5-to-10-minute walk to cool down

Tip: see if you can finish all this in under an hour!

Miss Mixalot

Coach Erica Coviello has made it through a million hard workouts and has assigned even more. There are two variations—one for intermediate to advanced marathoners, and one for beginning marathoners. This is an incredible workout if you want to strengthen your speed endurance. Your active recovery between tempo and mile pace is pretty short, which means you'll be digging in without feeling fully recovered during the work segments. Try doing this off the track to get a feel for running fast on the road.

Intermediate/Advanced Option

Run 1 mile at a slow pace and do the dynamic warm-up.

Run 2 miles at tempo pace.

Complete a 400-meter recovery jog.

Run 800 meters at mile pace.

Complete a 400-meter recovery.

Run 2 miles at tempo pace.

Cool down for 1 mile.

Beginner Option

This modified version is just half the distance at a quicker pace. It's good when you're short on time or not yet able to sustain tempo pace for two miles. Do this a time or two and you will likely be ready to hold that tempo for even longer.

Run 1 mile at a slow pace and do the dynamic warm-up.

Run 1 mile at tempo pace.

Complete a 400-meter recovery jog.

Run 400 meters at 15 seconds faster than mile pace.

Complete a 400-meter recovery.

Run 1 mile at tempo pace.

Cool down for 800 meters.

The Climb and Grind

This chapter would not be complete without a totally bonkers masterpiece of a workout from Coach Crystal. Find a fairly steep hill or jump on a treadmill. In terms of hill grade, 7 percent is ideal, but if you don't feel like doing math, scout an incline that is steeper than what you would consider rolling, but not as steep as the hill you use for hill sprints. It should be fairly long, enough to run uphill for a quarter mile. You'll want to run uphill at about a 10K pace and maintain a high-level effort until you reach the downhill recovery. If you're an advanced athlete, attempt this routine with minimal breaks.

> Run 1 slow mile.
>
> Run 400 meters uphill (aiming for about a 10K pace).
>
> Run another 400 meters at 5K pace. (If there's a flat surface at the top of the hill, that's ideal for this portion of the exercise—if not, continue uphill.) This is not a recovery!
>
> Do 10 squats.
>
> Do 10 jumping jacks.
>
> Do 10 reverse lunges.
>
> Do 10 burpees.
>
> Slowly jog downhill to where you started. If you are using a treadmill, run at a slow pace with no incline for about 90 seconds.
>
> Repeat for a total of 4 to 6 cycles.
>
> Complete a 1-mile cooldown.

GO RACE

I encourage every intermediate and advanced runner to sign up for a half-marathon "tune-up" race about midway through your in-season plan. For many marathoners, tucking a half-marathon into the training is the boost they need to finish the remaining weeks strong. It is a very effective dress rehearsal for your big race day. Plus, you can run relaxed, knowing that this race is just practice. You are essentially using it as a training run. It will give you insights into what you might need to work on. Maybe your fueling strategy isn't working when you run at race pace. Maybe you need to rethink your wardrobe choices. More likely than not, you will surprise yourself with the results. So many runners experience a breakthrough moment during tune-up races, because all the hard work they put in has paid off. They are quicker and fitter than in their wildest dreams.

IN THE GRIND

The first four weeks of in-season training will likely feel amazing and invigorating. The added running will give you an intense runner's high and let your serotonin and dopamine levels soar. Indeed, training often reduces anxiety and elevates mood. Running longer and crushing your goals just adds to this sensation. Cherish these feelings. Scan your body after those first four weeks and recognize just how fit you are.

Up until this point, the focus of training was on the build. Build muscles, build volume, build nutrition, build mental stamina. You have engineered yourself into a marathoner-in-training. Now it's time to fine-tune that progress. While the programming for beginners and advanced runners may look different, the goal is the same: you are training to make your engine bigger.

For beginner and intermediate runners, the early training periods helped establish a foundation on which we could build without compromising the structure. Now we can add some intensity so that you don't just finish, you finish feeling strong and running the time that is best for you. The in-season plans call for a slow progression of miles, weekly intense workouts, recovery days, and long runs. It should feel intense, especially when you enter the second month.

Advanced runners, the second month is the time to grind. By maximizing your weekly hard workouts, you will strengthen your force and potential. So while intermediate runners will encounter speedwork sessions that cap out at four miles, your plan will go beyond these relatively shorts sessions and may reach six miles of intervals, repeats, or tempos. In addition, your cooldown miles will increase to two or three miles following the workout. This will give you a chance to experience running on tired legs, mimicking what you will feel come race day. Race-pace and fartlek miles will be tucked into long runs. The plans in this guide do not go over twenty miles and do not recommend doing two twenty-mile runs in the same in-season cycle. Some coaches will recommend that advanced runners go longer than twenty on their long runs. But for the vast majority of amateur runners, taking on more than twenty miles offers more risk than reward. Besides, to rev up your engine, quality miles are going to matter far more than quantity.

The numbers on the plans and the specific workouts are all there for a reason—and that's to help you peak at just the right time. If you miss miles or skip a workout, don't try to make it up on a different day. Just move on. One workout is not going to make or break your run, but inserting random miles into the structure could throw the rest of your training off balance.

GRINDING TOO HARD

While the first four weeks of in-season training might feel incredible, like you are finally able to free the beast and train for your goal, after that point we must prepare for the physical and mental pitfalls that happen as your intensity and volume increase. At a certain point, generally when you hit the maximum number of weekly miles, your body might start to rebel. Some of this is totally normal, and there are solutions to ease the pain of the grind. Call it what you will—the middle-month struggle, the marathon blues—just know that it happens to plenty of runners who might find themselves asking, "Why am I doing this to myself again?" I've known plenty of runners who just stop at this point. Many of these runners were ill prepared. They might not have done the hard work to get to where you are right now. Others lost sight of their overall goals. You have to really want it, because by this point, the marathon will seep into just about every aspect of your life. Accept it and embrace that this is part of the journey! The latter part of this chapter will give you the motivation you need to keep crushing it if you do find yourself in a slump.

But if you're on week 3 or 4 and you're already feeling fatigued, stop for a beat. We have to make sure nothing more serious is going on with you physically. Or if the strain you're feeling in the max-load weeks is making it nearly impossible to get out of bed, then it is worthwhile to take a look at everything that's going on to ensure your health is OK. Too many people assume that because they are runners training for a marathon, they are in top physical condition. What's more accurate is that marathon training comes with great risks. Yes, it is generally beneficial to your well-being, but it can also cause some major problems. Before we get to how to deal with the common problems of marathon training, I think it's necessary to rule out more serious issues. Don't make the mistake of powering through serious symptoms and running yourself into the ground. So let's take a look at what's normal and what's not.

OVERUSE INJURIES AND OVERTRAINING SYNDROME

It's not normal to feel like you are in a constant fog, living in a nightmare where your muscles ache, you can't focus, your eyes won't stay open, and you want to sleep all day but can't relax. If you're experiencing symptoms like these or any other kind of overwhelming fatigue, a visit to your general practitioner or sports medicine doctor will help you sort out what's going on. It could be a few things. For instance, your brain might be overloaded by training. Maybe you're putting too much pressure on yourself and not focusing on self-care. Balancing life with training is freaking hard, and mental burnout is not something to be taken lightly. It's often accompanied by a shortage of sleep and poor eating, and can lead to physical health problems. If your stress level is too high, you will run tight, which will lead to a change in gait, which then leads to aches and pains, which may become injuries. That's an exhausting chain of events.

Dr. Jordan Metzl, also known as the Running Doctor, often says that 90 percent of runners he sees come to him during training. That means only 10 percent of runners injure themselves during the actual race. Most of the issues runners deal with are overuse. Aches in the Achilles tendon, hamstrings, calves, and feet might be slight at first but can lead to stress fractures, tendonitis, or shin splints. No matter the severity, they are all painful, and they are usually generated by too many miles too fast too soon.

If you can't see a doctor but you have a pain that is constant or keeps coming back after runs, it's probably worthwhile to ask yourself if it's being caused by running. Let's say, for example, I have a pain in my right shin. It is a dull, throbbing sensation when I'm walking or sitting. When I run, it feels like a nail is going through the bone in my right shin whenever my right foot strikes the ground. Those are classic shin splint symptoms, and shin splints are almost always caused by overuse. (They can also be caused by wearing ill-fitting shoes, so if this is happening to you, visit your local running shoe store and explain the pain to a shoe expert. They will look at your foot and find you something that will make you feel better.) The first thing to do when you suspect you have an overuse injury is to back off running. For shin splints, the constant pounding is what causes the pain. Don't give up on your training plan, though! Instead, take those miles to a bike, elliptical machine, or pool. It won't be exactly the same, but it will save you from developing a longer-lasting injury. After all, these little aches are your legs warning you to not do too much. Many sports doctors will tell you to rest for one to two weeks. That sounds like forever. But if you cross-train and continue your strength program, you'll come back to the plan even stronger.

Common Overuse Injuries in Running

Shin Splints

Also known as medial tibial stress syndrome, shin splints cause you pain along the tibia, the large bone in the front of your lower leg.

If you feel stabbing in your shins, assume it is shin splints. Follow RICE protocol:

Rest: Don't run for at least three days. Don't run if it still hurts.

Ice: Take an ice pack or a bag full of ice wrapped in a thin kitchen towel and apply it to the pain for fifteen minutes. If possible, do this three times per day.

Compression: Wrap the painful area in an Ace bandage or wear compression apparel. Think: those dorky high socks runners are always wearing.

Elevation: Try to keep the painful area elevated. This gives you a great excuse to put your feet up.

In addition to RICE, nonsteroidal anti-inflammatory medicines usually help. Go to a running-shoe store and make sure you have the right arch and ankle support in your running shoes. A change in shoes could literally make all the difference in your training.

Achilles Tendonitis

Your Achilles tendon is a band of tissue that connects your calf muscle to your lower leg. Runners get Achilles tendonitis from repeatedly extending the foot. You notice pain along your Achilles tendon, which travels down the leg. Don't be surprised if this flares up when you've gone longer than you have before.

RICE will help this condition. The other tried-and-true method to treat this is strengthening your calves and ankles with the stretches found earlier in this chapter (see page 147). Stretch and strengthen your calves, feet, and ankles.

Stress Fracture

Did you know that your bones constantly undergo a process called remodeling, where old bone tissue is removed and new bone tissue is rebuilt? I know, cool. Running strengthens your muscles and bones. But if you increase the intensity or duration of your running too quickly, your body can't keep up. It cannot generate new bone tissue fast enough for the remodeling process to be a success. This causes stress fractures, otherwise known as a runner's worst nightmare. In runners, the tibiae, hips, thighs, ankles, and feet are most often affected.

What does it feel like? A pain that just won't go away. Some people describe a crunching type of feeling. Stress fractures require more care than other common overuse injuries. Seriously, if this is something you are concerned about, stop running and go to the doctor.

Plantar Fasciitis

The most common complaint with plantar fasciitis is a stabbing pain in one or both heels. The condition involves irritation of the soft tissue band that runs along the bottom of your foot, which helps to support the arch. It often hurts the worst with the first steps of the day—when the plantar fascia is the tightest—and is worsened by running. Good news, though. Stretching (the arch stretch and big toe stretch) really will help this heal. It is best to stretch the tissue out first thing in the morning, before you even step out of bed. RICE will definitely help, but you likely won't need to take more than a few days off running if you catch it early and start a rehab protocol right away. If the pain lasts more than a few weeks, a podiatrist or your local running shop might be able to get you orthotics to better support your heel.

Overtraining Syndrome

Overtraining syndrome is a condition in which runners experience fatigue and declining performance despite continuing or increased training. While the overuse injuries I listed earlier are different from overtraining syndrome, these injuries can be a symptom of overtraining syndrome. Check out the list of symptoms below to know what to watch out for. If you're facing overtraining syndrome, you'll likely feel sluggish, unmotivated, and upset. Your RPE will be off the charts. Running is never supposed to feel so terrible that you dread the thought of putting on your running shoes. Athletes can develop overtraining syndrome long before they notice something is off. Unfortunately, runners often assume that they need to push through the pain, or they believe that seeing a doctor will bring their worst nightmare to fruition—they will have to take time off to heal. The very thought of not running, even if it is causing pain, can strike fear into many runners' hearts. But addressing complications early on can save your racing season. Ignore serious symptoms, and you could derail yourself for years.

So be in tune with your body. Refer back to this list anytime you suspect something is wrong. If you are experiencing three or more symptoms simultaneously, or if any number of symptoms is prohibiting you from living your life, close this book and schedule an appointment with your doctor. If you are cleared to run, then your next appointment should be with a coach.

Signs of Overtraining Syndrome

Exhaustion
Excessive hunger and thirst
Absence of appetite
Muscle fatigue
Numbness or tingling
Aches and pains
Injuries
Anxiety
Irritability
Elevated resting heart rate
Increased RPE
Colds or flu
Headaches
Changes to your menstrual cycle

A big problem with overtraining is the havoc it wreaks on your hormones. Your body starts producing too much of one thing and not enough of the other. You might get sick, or feel tired, or feel hungry all the time, or have no appetite at all. If your cortisol levels are either high or low, it can cause anxiety, sadness, or a general feeling of unease. Overtraining can also cause thyroid problems, which might present as extreme tiredness; anxiety; strange body sensations like being cold all the time, numbness, or tingling; and disrupted sleep.

Finally, if your menstrual cycle gets out of whack, then you know your body is in distress. Some women have a change in the duration of their flow, or they lose their period completely, while others experience terrible PMS thanks to plummeting progesterone. While some hormonal changes are inevitable and benign, every woman should know what the female athlete triad is and what it looks like. The American College of Obstetricians and Gynecologists defines it as a medical condition caused by an overexpenditure of energy observed in physically active females involving three components:

1. Low energy availability with or without disordered eating
2. Menstrual dysfunction
3. Low bone density

Though it's called a triad, you do not need to have all three symptoms to be diagnosed. Most commonly, the first symptom women will pay attention to is a missed or irregular period. It's a common misconception that women who are extremely thin are the only people who can be affected by this disease; every body type is susceptible. If you think you might be experiencing female triad syndrome, contact a doctor right away. Even if you are miraculously able to train and compete at a high level with this disorder, it can cause reproductive problems and osteoporosis later on in life.

IT'S JUST THE BLUES

If you are certain that the issue is not physical, then perhaps you're experiencing the "marathon blues." This is a slump that comes along with massive mileage gains. Some of the symptoms of marathon blues include:

1. Being hungry most of the time (this might include experiencing cravings for things like Twinkies, soda, fries, doughnuts, and other sweet or greasy goodness)
2. Feeling more tired than usual
3. Aches, pains, and stiffness
4. General grumpiness

If you are in the midst of the marathon blues, then please know that I feel your pain. The middle weeks might make you feel like a hot mess. Everything is a struggle. First, if you are compulsively talking about your marathoning, don't stop. Let those words flow, girl. Like I said before, the training pervades every aspect of your life, and you should be proud of everything you're accomplishing. Your friends and family will embrace it and want to know everything. The random guy at the coffee shop doesn't mind listening for a second. Your coworkers will need to know why you are eating all the time, falling asleep in meetings, and walking like your muscles are on fire, so brag away.

The cold, hard truth of the matter is that this portion of training is really uncomfortable. Not only do you have tiredness, hunger, and physical aches to deal with, but you might be more emotional than usual. While some of this is unavoidable (hey, it's all making you stronger!), there are some things you can do to make the marathon blues a little less intense. And if you're in a really bad pit of despair but not quite at the point of needing medical attention, then making a plan of action with the following information is essential to keep you moving along:

1. Track your food. This might be the only time I ever tell anyone to count calories. Are you consuming what you need? Are your protein needs in line with your activity level and weight? Are you consuming enough carbohydrates and fats? Can you cut back on sugars that might be causing ups and downs? Refer to chapter 8 to ensure that you are eating enough. It is very possible that you're not eating enough!
2. Track your hydration. Ensure that you are getting enough minerals and electrolytes.

3. Track your sleep. How many hours are you getting? Is it restful? Did you dream?
4. Track your heart rate.

If you are finding some cracks in the foundation, then now is the time to patch them. It is far better to realize that you aren't eating enough weeks before race day than it is to look back weeks after the race and realize that you failed your body by essentially starving it for days on end. In addition, paying attention to the details will allow you to see if your body is recovering properly. You can adjust your training schedule accordingly.

For example, let's say that you are scheduled to run an 8 x 800 repeat workout. If you wake up on that day and record that you did not sleep well and your resting heart rate is higher than usual, you should recognize that your rest and recovery leading up to that workout is not on point. That's OK; that happens for about a billion reasons. But if you're feeling crappy already, don't feel like you need to push and push and push to force yourself to complete the workout. Consider altering what's on your plan. Run 4 x 800. Run three easy miles instead. Or take a three-mile walk and mindfully hydrate.

My former colleague Meghan Kita uses common sense when it comes to training. Meghan is a Pennsylvania-based RRCA running coach and the author of *How to Make Yourself Poop: And 999 Other Tips Every Runner Should Know*, though she may be best known as the woman who broke the Guinness World Record for fastest female marathoner dressed as fast food (a hot dog). Her best advice for all marathoners? Don't be a slave to the plan. Taking an unscheduled rest day does not make you less of a runner. Sometimes it's actually better if you take the time to let your muscles and heart rest. You will come back and crush the next workout and feel great doing it. Unless you take fourteen days off, you will not lose any fitness. Give yourself the time and space you need. Recharge, refresh, and replenish instead of turning yourself into a dumpster fire.

SET SMART GOALS

If you have tracked all you can track and found that there is nothing physically out of whack, then the issue might stem from boredom, mental exhaustion, or feeling overwhelmed. This is natural—training for a marathon is a long and massive undertaking.

In this case, I want you to take a moment each week to make SMART training goals. SMART is a mnemonic that stands for specific, measurable, attainable, relevant, time-based.

This is really different from your intrinsic goals, which are used for overall motivation and inspiration. Your weekly SMART goals give you something to work toward and achieve.

Let's say I keep skipping the dynamic warm-up, even though I know it's important. My SMART goal for week one can be "Complete the dynamic warm-up before five workouts by Saturday."

Now let's say that setting a goal like that makes training feel even more like a chore and adds to my general malaise. My next SMART goal should be something more lighthearted that could give me a glimpse of ultimate marathon success. Maybe I try this: "Add a race-pace mile into Tuesday's six-miler."

When I've talked to marathoners who have experienced the blues, there's a common denominator in their suffering: they've lost sight of everything they've accomplished and just how much work they have put in. Every single goal, every workout, every long run, everything is a reason to celebrate. If you want to buy yourself flowers or balloons, you should. But just giving yourself a small pat on the back every time you complete another daily run goes a long way in keeping motivation high.

AMP IT UP

Sometimes, though, no amount of positivity or goal setting can make you feel fresh and new. But keeping your schedule interesting can break you free from the doldrums of marathon training.

Make It a Destination

Plan a staycation around your long run. Find a nearby town and map out your route. If you have the resources and time, grab a reservation at a hotel. Finish your run, shower, and treat yourself to a nice brunch at a new-to-you restaurant. By planning your long run and making it special, you take the focus off the training itself and make the miles something to experience with a reward at the end.

Run a Local 5K

There is nothing that gets a runner's happiness level up like a local race. To see people of all levels lining up at the start and to be part of that crowd, man, it's so special. Racing is a great reminder of how lucky we are that we get to run alongside one another. There is nothing quite like the feeling of being at the start of the race, no matter how big or small. So yes, it will boost your mood. Find a weekend race in your area. If you're a beginning marathoner, running a few shorter races while you train will help your mind prep for marathon morning. Run the 5K slowly, and then do the rest of your long run immediately after. If you are an intermediate or advanced runner, you can race the 5K or run it as a tempo, then finish your long run.

Go Point to Point

I don't know why, but when I am in a funk, I hate running a loop or an out-and-back. I want to start in one place and end somewhere new. During one training cycle, I asked my husband to drive behind me so I could leave one of our cars at the Valley Forge Park in Pennsylvania. We then drove together to the Perkiomen trailhead. We got out and ran eighteen miles back to the other car. Just getting to somewhere else lifted my spirits. It made me think, "Wow, look at how many miles I covered. Look where I can get myself to!"

Find Friends

Sometimes all you need are friends to share the suckiness with you. When you run with other people, you have the chance to gossip, compare notes, and talk about things that aren't running, and all of this takes your mind off the task at hand. If you don't have friends who run, head to your local running store and ask if there are any groups or clubs in your area. You will be placed with people in your same pace range, and I promise, runners are talkers. You are destined to make new friends.

JUST DO IT

You know, sometimes there simply isn't much you can do. If you feel really burned out and running sucks and things in life keep dragging you down, give yourself permission to feel like doggy doo-doo. Training will be a beast sometimes, and you don't always have to shift your perspective or pretend to be happy. Don't wallow in it, but don't get mad when you feel drained or grumpy. Marathoning takes a ton of mental and physical energy, so you are not going to feel like a magical sunflower all the time.

Speaking of magical flowers, I asked my BFF, Hannah McGoldrick, what she does when she gets the marathon blues. Her advice? Get through those terrible weeks. Know that there is a light at the end of the tunnel. By the time she runs her goal race, she's long forgotten that she ever felt that way. And usually hours after she crosses the finish line, she signs up for another marathon.

In-season training is no joke, and it just continues to get harder until three weeks before the race, which is when you cut back on miles to prime your body for race day. In the next chapter, we will make your determination bulletproof, so that no mental block will get in your way during these tough training days.

CHAPTER 10

YOU ARE TOUGH ENOUGH

By now, you probably know about the little glitches in your body—the not-so-serious but super annoying aches that appear at mile six and stay with you for the duration of your long runs. You've identified your weaknesses, and maybe you're even working on them. But for so many runners, the number one thing that holds them back from their true potential is mental.

First we'll learn how to embrace the pain, so to speak. Next we'll focus on the mental blocks that get runners down. There are strategies to practice, ways to cope, and a number of reframing techniques and positivity practices to propel you to the finish line.

Until this point, I told you to focus any visualization techniques and imagery sessions on your training. That hyperfocus on the preparation should have, in a perfect world, improved your running economy, given you confidence, and helped you to feel comfortable letting your body do the work while the mind was quiet. Sticking to a mental training plan is hard, I know. So if this element of your preparation hasn't been a priority, I understand. Now is the time to get your head back in the game.

There is so much more than gaining running experience that you can do to mentally prepare for the feat you are about to accomplish. Can you make it through the marathon on pure determination and a no-quit attitude? Yeah, you can. I have relied on that method for many races. But I credit many of my PRs to using some of these mind techniques. The good news is, no matter where you are in your mental practice, there are ways to prepare for race day.

GET OVER EVERY WALL

I've said it before, and I'll say it again. Marathon training is hard. Running a marathon is hard. If you're trying to push yourself to meet a specific time goal, it's going to be even harder. The best thing you can do to mentally prepare yourself for this reality is to accept it.

Now, that doesn't mean you should psych yourself out. I said it will be hard—not impossible! On the opposite end of the spectrum, trying to convince yourself that it will be easy could be even more detrimental. There's an old adage that's passed from old-school runners to new generations: "Respect the distance." Know that at times this training and this distance will try to defeat you.

You won't be defeated, though. Not by the training as a whole, a specific workout, or the race. We've already gone over how to test your strengths and use them to build confidence. And we know how to practice getting in the zone.

You might have heard runners talk about "hitting the wall." If you physically hit the wall, it means your glycogen stores are depleted and your body is struggling to find energy, and this shouldn't happen if your fueling plan is dialed in. More commonly, runners hit a mental wall. Maybe your legs begin to feel like concrete, and you're panting, and you can't stop thinking about how uncomfortable you are inside your own skin. A 2008 study compared the minds of elite runners and amateur runners during the marathon and looked specifically at when runners hit the wall. It found that the elite runners were able to tune in to what was happening to their bodies. Amateurs, however, "purposely tried to cut themselves off from the sensory feedback they would normally receive from their body during the run."

What does that mean exactly? Elite athletes possess the knowledge, training, and ability it takes to stay in an uncomfortable physical and/or mental state. In some instances, an elite athlete can identify the trouble area and use psychological techniques to reduce the intensity of the feeling. Meanwhile, runners who run on the "just get through it" method might try to ignore the pain or disassociate from what is going on inside the body or even in their outer surroundings. If you've ever tried to do this, you know that denying the terribleness that is happening only makes the sensation stronger. No amount of praying will take the pain away. Like I said, you can make it to the finish line by sheer determination. But all that denial wastes energy, and believe it or not, there are ways to think your way through a tough spot. Here's how:

1. Accept the Pain

OK, so you feel like you're dying and you can't go on. The first thing to do is acknowledge that pain and name it. What is one word to describe your physical state? Maybe you're tired, nauseated, overheated. What is one word to describe your mental state? This could be *anxious, frustrated, annoyed,* or *bored.* Let yourself feel these things. Every moment of the run doesn't have to be incredible. There are times when it really sucks, and you know what? That's good. That means you are testing yourself and doing hard things. If you feel like crying, cry. If you feel like letting out a grunt, a yelp, a scream, let it out. Sometimes emitting some sort of noise frees you of tension and lets you harness your inner power. Don't be alarmed if you aren't feeling like the best you. So you're having a rough mile. Feel it, live it, release it. Remind yourself that all the things you are feeling will soon pass. They will pass, and you will feel stronger than before.

2. Breathe Through It

First, change the pattern of your breath. If you were breathing in on your left foot first, change it to your right. Take a big belly breath in, and blow it out hard through pursed lips. Simply getting back in touch with your breath and taking in more oxygen can renew your spirit. If that is not enough, or your breath is ragged and out of control, slow down. Shake out your arms and loosen your shoulders. Do a body scan and name the things that are bothering you. You should feel empowered to walk if you need to, because you will be able to return to a normal pace after you get over this hump. Once your body scan is complete and you've identified your trouble spots, isolate each area you need to focus on. If your legs feel heavy, breathe that heavy feeling up from your calves through your chest to your nostrils and release it in a big, open-mouthed exhale. With your next inhale, send a cold breath to the legs. Repeat this a few times.

3. Find Mindfulness

Many people think that mindfulness is some sort of state of nirvana, but it's really not anything fancy. It's the ability to just be. You've been mindful about what's bothering you; now it's time to turn outward and be present in the run. Look at your surroundings. What is around you? Name five things you see and five things you hear. What do you smell? What do you taste? What does it sound like? Are you on an empty road? Is it peaceful? When I'm trying to make myself present in the run, I will pretend I'm high-fiving trees so I can experience the tactile sensation of my fingers touching the branches. Weird? Yes, I mean, I could pay attention to my feet on the pavement or my arms swishing by my sides, and all that would be just fine. But you need to find what works and what doesn't.

4. Inspire Yourself

Call your intrinsic goal to mind both when you're running with ease and when you're slogging through your miles. Remember back when you set this goal in chapter 1? Calling it to mind while you're training will only strengthen your bond with what you want to accomplish and make you feel like you are truly achieving whatever that *why* is. It's so easy to get sucked into the drudgery of following a plan, pounding out miles, focusing on the race and nothing else. So please, remember to take a second and remember your *why* during runs. It will make the physical exertion feel so much easier.

....

It might be hard to employ these things at will during a race if you haven't tried them in your training. Not every run will be good. If you are struggling on a long run, and you know it's a mental block, enlist these tools. To become a master of your mind, try them on any kind of run—when you feel good, when you are tired, on short runs, on hard runs, even when you are strength training. The more you build the mind-body connection, the better you will handle whatever comes up on race day.

DEVELOPING GRIT

What is grit? Where does it come from? For some, it means having heart, never giving up, running to the best of your ability to the very end. For others, it means rising above challenges. As runners, we test ourselves every single day. Every mile is an accomplishment and proves our tenacity. Maybe some people are born with grit, but most grinders I know worked through tough times and learned to apply their never-give-up attitude to everything they do. I know a lot of runners like that.

In marathoning, grit is something we want to cultivate and expand. You will need determination to the point of stubbornness to make it through a whole training cycle and achieve your race dreams. All you have to do is know and celebrate your worth. Every single runner has the capacity to conquer her goals. If doubt ever creeps in, crush it immediately, because you can handle anything.

Every week you follow the plan builds a stronger foundation. Of course, with all the effort you put forth, there will be days when you are mentally exhausted. There will be some runs where you feel like you cannot take another step. When this happens, I want you to draw on all the runs you've done to this point. If you're on your eighth four hundred repeat out of twelve, close your eyes and visualize the last time you completed a track workout. You've been here before; you can make it to the end again. These runs, the ones that feel impossible but that you push yourself through, will be the workouts you can think about on race day when things get hard. You are tenacious. You are confident, and you are prepared.

THE BLOCKS

Negative emotions are part of marathoning. But left unchecked, these bothersome thoughts can actually prevent flow state and mess with your race performance. Think of that chatterbox ego that likes to pick apart every run. It is really common that our minds conjure up the ghosts of old anxieties the closer we get to race day. And race day itself? Forget it. Unless you're an alien, you're going to feel nervous.

But do not fear! In her book, *Don't Leave Your Mind Behind: The Mental Side of Performance*, Nicole Detling, PhD, CMPC, discusses the role anxiety plays in performance. You've likely already experienced prerace jitters. You can expect the same butterflies in your stomach and that annoying constant urge to pee at just about every start line. Detling, and a large number of sports psychologists, would tell you to take that tiny bit of nervousness and use it to your advantage.

Instead of saying, "I'm so nervous," try saying, "I'm so excited." Start saying this now. Fighting the anxiousness is self-defeating, and those nervous feelings are so closely related to excitement that it only makes sense to channel them into the adrenaline that will already be pumping through you when you get to the start.

Being nervous is a good thing! It means you're invested and you're awake. If you're feeling this before the proverbial gun goes off, go through your visualization routine and hold on to that extra energy. Get ready to use it when you need it.

But sometimes our nerves can run amok. A lot of that has to do with timing. If you've raced before and you know that you start to feel a strange worrying sensation days before you get to the start line, that's not ideal. You don't want to waste time or mental space trying to deal with this. And believe me, I've been there. I talked to a collegiate athlete who, before seeking help, would be so anxious a week from a race that she would shake uncontrollably and sometimes feel like she was going to throw up.

Thought stopping will help. And indeed, many of the breathing and reframing tips in this book can help with the kind of anxiety that shows up and lingers for weeks. And of course, consulting a therapist or sports psychologist is your best bet. They can help you take back control over a multitude of negative emotions.

But you can get a head start by slowing down and analyzing the anxiety you feel. Ask yourself:

What am I actually nervous about?
Where does this come from?
Could it possibly be tied to fear?
Now ask yourself this question: Why? What am I afraid of?

The answer to the last question is essential for you to identify. Because seriously, what is actually at stake? Some people might realize that the worst thing they can imagine happening isn't that bad. Or you might feel like your fear might really be devastating. That's OK. You don't have to push it out of your mind or try to convince yourself that it won't happen. Instead, you can reason with this fear. Often, when we're able to examine our fears closely, we realize that we're more than capable of handling them.

You can say: "OK, some things are out of my control and might prevent me from reaching all my goals on race day. But I am as prepared as I can be. No matter what happens, I will have succeeded in making it through a tough training process. I am really strong and fit." Now let's break down a few different types of fear. It's the best way to face it and get over it.

Fear of Disaster

Some runners go through a string of terrible and paranoid thoughts leading up to race day. These ideas are very often based on things out of your control.

For example, what if there's a tornado in the middle of the race? What if my foot explodes? What if I simultaneously throw up and poop my pants and can't finish? What if I suffer dehydration? What if I get lost? What if a rabid raccoon tackles me?

These examples are extreme, but if you're doing this annoying "what if" thing during training, it's no good. Thinking like this will literally drain your energy. Whenever your mind starts going on like that, picture a stop sign. Just stop. If that's too jarring, try to picture the words in your head, and then imagine them exploding like fireworks. This is a little cognitive behavioral therapy technique that helps conquer obsessive negative thoughts. Give it a shot.

Remember, you can control only what is in your control. You are prepared, and if Mother Nature decides to drop a tornado on your marathon, then so be it. You will achieve your dream at another race.

Fear of the Unknown

I know a runner named Amy who is one of the most determined and intelligent people I know. When she signed up for her first marathon, she was psyched through her whole training. Nothing got her down. I was impressed by her commitment to the plan and her positive attitude. Until she got to the taper, which is the final two weeks before the race, when you back off training duration and intensity. In her training bliss, Amy hardly saw the taper coming. It was like she suddenly opened her eyes and saw that her race was two weeks away. She called me the morning after her Saturday run, which was longish (like twelve miles). This is a normal long run when you're that close to your race. She was perplexed, she said. I asked her why.

"Well, I'm two weeks away from running a race, I am decreasing my mileage, but I've only gone for twenty miles."

"Right?" I didn't know what the problem was. She'd had a near-perfect training cycle.

"Shouldn't I have run the full 26.2 at some point?"

"No plan goes up that high." You all know by now that running anything close to the full distance before the race just isn't worth the risk of injury. But then it dawned on me: a first-time marathoner might want to know what those extra miles will feel like. I remember ignoring the ten-mile cutoff and going a full thirteen when I ran my first half-marathon, just to assure myself that I could handle the extra time. I didn't need to do that. Physically, I was ready. That's what I told Amy. Calm down, I said. You're ready and you've got this. You put in the work, and once you get to the last six miles, you'll have run twenty already—what an accomplishment! Nothing will be able to stop you.

Here's what you need to know. There is no way to predict how your race will go. The entire 26.2 miles will be unknown because no two miles are ever the same. How exhilarating is that? So the last six? You have to trust yourself, trust your plan, trust your body, and let go of any hesitation.

Fear of Failure

When you ask yourself what you're afraid of and the answer is something like "I might not finish" or "I don't want to run a bad time," then you're not alone. These are common thoughts and it's OK to feel some amount of apprehension. After all, you spend a lot of time preparing for one day, and you want it to be your best showing.

The problem with this fear is that it often results in trying too hard to prevent whatever failure we feel is lurking. Trying too hard means running tight. Running tight means depleted energy.

It might not assuage your fear, but you will finish. And when you finish, even if the time on the clock doesn't show the number you want, it's still a good time.

If for some reason you don't finish, and if you don't meet your extrinsic goals, it is not the end of the world. Maybe it wasn't your day. Remember, making it to the start line is the real feat. The amount of dedication and training you put in is a testament to your strength. The finish line is the cherry on top— and if you fail, you will recover and return to racing with lessons learned.

You might not be able to control everything that happens in the race, so don't be hard on yourself. You have already come so far.

NO MORE SELF-DOUBT

Sometimes negative self-talk morphs into self-doubt, which will absolutely disrupt your race. Self-doubt is kind of sneaky and might appear even when you're doing everything right. It might visit in the middle of the race. It often comes in the form of a question: I'm running such a great pace right now. Can I keep it up? I am feeling stronger than I ever have, but is this for real? Can I do this? Can I finish?

I'm telling you from personal experience, those nagging little "can I" statements creep their way into your subconscious and slow you down. The problem with self-doubt is that it disguises itself as a rational thought. So you listen, and you might think you're being pragmatic. I always thought I was being realistic and trying my best not to set myself up for disappointment. One day, during my second marathon training cycle, I sat down to eat lunch with a fast friend. She asked me how my training was going. I mentioned that I was feeling very strong, and so I was worried that I was peaking too early.

To me, this seemed like a valid concern. Never before had I made it through a sixteen-miler with such ease.

"Did you ever think that you're improving?" she said.

No! Of course I had never considered that. That type of clearheaded positive thinking would be very off-brand for me.

"You have to think about this in a different way," she said. "Otherwise that neurosis will turn into a self-fulfilling prophecy."

I knew she was right. A lot of us let those doubtful thoughts flood our brain because we're scared. Scared that we can't achieve any of our (usually extrinsic) goals. (See, fear strikes again!)

I asked the sports psychologist and running coach Kirstin Ritchie what we are supposed to do with self-doubt. Coach Kirstin has run six marathons, including two Boston Marathons and two sub-three-hour finishes, with a 2:57 PR at the 2016 Hartford Marathon. Still, she understands the annoying self-doubt that can creep into any athlete's mind.

"The main thing is to reaffirm that you're actually capable and draw on actual evidence to support that," she says. "A lot of times, you limit yourself by what you believe you're capable of."

But if we just let ourselves relax and run, we would be more than capable. When you hear yourself asking questions that sound like self-doubt, rephrase them into "I am" statements.

> Can I sustain this pace? → This pace feels comfortable. I am strong.
> Am I training right? → I am following the plan and doing every-
>   thing right. I am improving.
> Am I ready? → I trust myself and the process. I am ready.
> Can I finish? → I am ready and excited to finish.
> Can I do it? → I am capable.

If you have different annoying questions that could lead to self-doubt, try reworking them here:

_____ → _____

_____ → _____

_____ → _____

IMAGINE RACE DAY

Whether or not you're struggling with negative emotions, the key to increasing the chance of flow state is in the meditative practice of imagery. You have successfully imagined various training scenarios, and you can see yourself from a third-person point of view and also view the world from a first-person perspective. Now is the time to shift your imagery sessions to race-day scenarios.

There is some prep work involved to create the ideal visualization. If you live close to your racecourse, take the time to look at the race map, see where each mile is, and take mental snapshots of any features of the course that stand out to you. Choose easy-to-remember locations like the start, the finish, the halfway point, a hill you love to hate, a cool tree. It should be a mixture of things that you think will be a challenge and things that will bring you joy.

If you don't live near your race destination, then your visualizations might require a bit more imagination. Do a Google image search of your race and try to match various locations with the course map. Some races might have video of the course online. And if your race has a Facebook page, you can ask locals about landmarks or sections you might need to know about. Seriously, your best resource will always be other runners. No matter what you find, you should include the start and finish in your sessions.

The first time you use the imagery for race day, bring up the snapshot of the start line. If you can, populate the area around you with other runners. Try to hear the music blaring. Feel your toes in your shoes. Feel your excitement building, your blood getting hot. You are moments from taking off. Jump up and down once. Notice what you are wearing, paying attention to each piece of your outfit. Picture it and also notice how it feels. Are you carrying anything? Smell and feel the air around you. Then open your eyes.

The important part of bringing the start line into view is preparing yourself for that moment. In future sessions, try to feel any emotions that arise. They might vary. That's fine because it will prepare you for whatever comes up on race day.

The goal is to cycle through each of the visual snapshots you took of the course and imagine them as scenarios in various imagery sessions. If you think a particular feature will be challenging, you may want to spend extra time working through it in your mind. Remember to use your differing points of view. If you want to envision yourself using perfect form, try the third person. If you want to intentionally introduce confidence into the scene, use first person.

At the end of this book, there is another imagery prompt that can be used as a guide the night before the big day. Achieving flow state is ideal, but even if you can't get totally in the zone on race day, using these exercises will help your mind and body relax and focus.

The other thing to recognize is what the process of training gives to you. While it's important to harness the power of your emotions, recognize the incredible strength that training for this monumental distance has instilled in you. Your dedication and sacrifices to this distance have made you a more determined and overall incredible human. Not everyone can handle this task. Remember just how amazing you are, not just on race day but every day.

CHAPTER 11

THE TAPER

About three weeks before race day, you will start to taper. The taper is when you start decreasing your mileage in order to give your body an opportunity to rest and recover before the big day. Enjoy this period. Know that all the hard work is behind you and it will pay off once you reach the finish line. If this is your first rodeo, you might be looking at your training plan and asking if the coach who made it is out of her mind. You'll notice a significant drop in mileage and basically no hard-effort runs.

Most coaches and plans will have you cut weekly mileage volume by 20 to 30 percent each week from your highest-volume week, for three weeks. That first week of the taper won't feel too different. Your body will just think, "Oh, cool, it's a cut-down week." Then comes the next week. In comparison to that forty-mile week you ran in the grind of training, you will feel like you're not running at all.

Hopefully, this little break before the big day is a welcome reprieve. After all, there is a scientific benefit to cutting back in the last fourteen days. It should be noted, however, that these days of rest will come with some, well, trials of their own. It's best to prep yourself for what experienced marathoners call the Taper Tantrums. These weeks have the tendency to bring out a lot of emotions and some oddities. I should also mention that not everyone experiences the Taper Tantrums—I never fear the taper, so if you're like me, and you are super pumped to run two miles and then nap, thank goodness! You are trusting your training, and girl, you have got this. But if you notice that you're freaking out during this time, know that it happens to many marathoners, and read on.

So why do we do it? Why not just keep slogging along, building and building until we reach race day? We taper because the body needs rest! During the two- or three-week taper, there is some cool stuff going on inside your body. Your muscles and tendons, which have been working overtime and going through the process of getting worn down, finally have an opportunity to rebuild and strengthen. Your hormones level out. Metabolic enzymes and antioxidants return to their optimal ranges. All of this is in preparation for an epic performance. Some studies indicate a 3 percent improvement in performance in people who tapered compared with people who attempted to stick to a rigorous training schedule all the way up until the big day.

It sounds like common sense, and yet I hear the question all the time: Do I really need to taper? The answer is, unequivocally, yes. Listen up: tapering is one of the most important parts of marathon training.

First, you might get it in your head that because you're not running as many miles, you're not really working. Like I said before, your body is actually working overtime to prepare you to run your best 26.2 miles. Despite not running a full load, you must continue to focus on your nutrition, hydration, and overall well-being. In fact, this is the time to really dial it in. Don't change too much, but try to hydrate the right amount. Continue to consume the same number of calories and include more carbs. Don't get discouraged if you feel a little bloated. That's actually good! It means you're re-upping your glycogen stores. You will burn it all on race day. And if I catch you on the scale, I will hunt you down and scream. Yeah, you might gain a pound or two. Guess what? You will end up losing five to eight pounds during the course of the marathon. (You'll also shrink, on average, about one centimeter because your spine gets compressed. Cool, right? Don't worry, you will bounce right back to your normal height within twenty-four hours.) Get enough sleep, but don't laze around in bed. Take short walks and stretch your body out. Be good to yourself.

Finally, pay attention to intensity. The plans in this book have two hard efforts included in the taper. Don't listen to people who tell you to do Yasso eight hundreds to predict your time. I love Yasso eight hundreds, but man, those are for earlier in the season. Do not go out and do a long hill workout. Don't listen to the other extreme, our conservative friends who urge you to stick to easy miles. There is a perfect middle ground that will keep your body primed without depleting you and compromising your recovery before the race, and that's the plan outlined in the in-season training plan.

A COMPREHENSIVE GUIDE TO NOT LOSING IT

The experienced marathoner might've learned to dread the taper period and might've made up her mind to skip it altogether and train as usual. That's not a good look. A great number of runners refuse to taper because of fear—they're afraid that if they stop training, they will lose their fitness or come out flat on race day.

I promise, and experts agree, you will not gain anything by training hard in the last fourteen days before a race! You put in the work already, our bodies need six weeks at minimum to make lasting gains, and you don't need to do more. At this point, you don't have enough time to make any improvements by running. You do have the chance to refresh yourself and replenish your energy stores. Harness the power you have and enjoy the fitness you've created up to this point.

Trust yourself. Trust your mind, your legs, your feet and every other part of your body that is regenerating itself right now. In fact, this is the moment to thank your body for getting you this far and to engage in some much-needed self-care.

Whenever you find yourself wanting to run more miles than what's on your training plan, choose an item from this self-care list.

1. Shower or bathe.
2. Foam-roll for ten minutes.
3. Stretch for ten minutes.

4. Write a running-related gratitude list, trying to get to fifty.
5. Do a beauty treatment, if you're into that kind of thing.
6. Give yourself a pedicure. Choose a dark color that will cover up those bruised and broken toenails. Note: do not scrub off your runner's calluses. You earned those and they prevent blisters!
7. Ice any aches for fifteen to twenty minutes, alternating with heat.
8. Prepare and eat something delicious and nutritious.
9. Practice race-day visualization.
10. Write out ten things about yourself that are awesome.
11. Call a running buddy.
12. Take a mindfulness walk.

In addition to these suggestions, I want you to really pay attention to how your runs feel during the taper. First-time marathoners might take on a weekend twelve-miler and find themselves confused at the finish, asking, "I'm done already?" Intermediate and advanced runners: Take a physical and mental inventory each time you hit the road. Do a body scan and be mindful of how easy these runs feel to you now. Yes, the taper is the home stretch, but don't get hyperfocused on the future. Instead, take each day and each run as it comes. Enjoy your newfound strength. Feel your legs, arm, core, and breath as they get stronger during these weeks. You did the work and now your body is working for you.

YOU MIGHT GET ANGSTY

During the taper, new anxiety might creep in. Fun, right? Because you're running less, you'll have more time to dwell on those terrible "what ifs." First, remember what I told you in chapter 7 about disrupting those obnoxious thoughts. Practice some thought stopping, girl! If those what-if thoughts are accompanied by a feeling of restlessness or butterflies in your stomach and it's a little uncomfortable, first, know that this is very common. Second, I want you to do two things:

1. Every time this happens, close your eyes and imagine yourself taking the first step of the race. Repeat this statement: "I am so excited. I can't wait to race." This mini visualization only needs to last for ten seconds. What we're doing is channeling any nervous energy into a reserve of excitement. On race morning, you will be able to dip into that even after the initial adrenaline wears off. If the thought "I am nervous" enters your brain, that's OK. You're allowed to be nervous. You've made it so far. But then ask what you're nervous about. Is it anything you can control? Are you also really pumped to get to the start line? Yeah, I thought so! Reframing nervousness and anxiety into something more positive will make that tension melt away.

2. Breathe. The best breathing to calm down is square breathing. Not to sound like the world's most anxious person, but I practice square breathing no less than ten times a day. And I do it at every single start line. To do it, take a big belly breath in for four counts and hold for four counts. Release slowly for four counts, then hold for four counts. Repeat as needed.

3. If you're still feeling anxious after visualizing and breathing, watch something funny. This sounds simple, but laughing interrupts the anxiety response in the body.

YOU MIGHT FEEL STRANGE

One of the strangest things that people experience during the taper period is the phenomenon of phantom injuries. I promise you, I am not making this up. A runner will go out on a slow and easy run during the last week before the race and feel something that resembles pain. Maybe it's a tickle or an ache or just something different from how that body part is supposed to feel, and all of a sudden, you are certain that your entire body is going to spontaneously combust.

During her taper period, a friend of mine complained to me that she had a sudden onset of shin splints. This friend (a real neurotic to the core, which is why we get along) is an advanced runner who'd excelled in her training and was possibly in the best shape of her running life. The pain, she told me, was bilateral and shot up and down from her ankles to her knees. It did not hurt enough to stop her, and in fact, it was just a dull ache, but it was weird. "Why is this happening now?" she asked, nearly in tears. I had no idea. I didn't doubt that she felt the pain. I said to get to a doctor ASAP, and she did.

The doctor cleared her to run the race but advised her to take it easy in the days leading up to it. There was no stress fracture, no bruising, no lumps on her shinbones. If it was shin splints, the doc wasn't sure why it was happening now. She was a seasoned athlete who trained conservatively. Was it her shoes? Had she changed them recently? No. Were they flat? Did she need new ones? She didn't think so.

After the race, my pal told me that the pain in her legs dulled by the second mile. By the time she crossed the finish line, the aching had disappeared. Other parts of her body hurt, sure, but not the mystery shin splints. Her physical therapist told her after the race that it might've been psychosomatic—stress and fear manifested in the form of physical pain. Is that science? I don't think so. But this occurs in a great number of runners. It's important to note that she did everything right in this situation. She consulted her doctor and PT to make sure it wasn't anything serious, she rested her legs, and she rejoiced when the mysterious injury vanished.

PREDICT THE WEATHER

Some experts and coaches might tell you to not check the weather obsessively. I know that my coach has told me to look at it two days out, then one day out, then race morning, just to know if I need to change my outfit or rain gear or an extra pair of socks. These coaches are wise. You can't control it, they say, so why worry about it? It's true. You literally have no control over what Mother Nature decides to dish out that day. But are these coaches human beings or androids? Who can help obsessing about something as fickle as the weather? What I've found in my own racing adventures is that wanting to check the weather and then stopping myself creates more worry. Check the dang weather. If you need to cry about a predicted blizzard on your May race day, then cry. Then add more layers to your race outfit. If the weather changes each time you check it, then make a special place for all the gear you may or may not need. It can be your little marathon shrine of outfit options.

OVERPREPARE

During the taper, I like to make race checklists. I write out a preparation list for the days leading up to the marathon, and then I do a race-morning list. Here's an example, but keep in mind everyone's will be different because everyone is their own unique runner.

Taper Checklist

○ **14 days:** Print race map and directions. Go over them. Start a folder for this checklist, any gratitude, affirmation, or mantra lists you have, and all the other printouts you may need for race day.

○ **13 days:** Go over parking, shuttle service, or public transportation. If traveling, confirm hotel room and airline ticket.

○ **10 days:** Search for restaurants and menus near where the race is for a postrace feast, and make reservations.

○ **9 days:** Pack a suitcase and/or race bag:

> Race essentials:
> ☐ Fuel
> ☐ Water bottle
> ☐ Sunscreen
> ☐ Sunglasses
> ☐ Outfit
> ☐ Shoes
> ☐ Socks + extras
> ☐ Extra safety pins

○ **8 days:** Make an epic race playlist and two backups, plus a psych-up playlist that is equal parts motivational and soothing, for that time period while you are standing at the start waiting to take off.

○ **5 days:** Go over arrival at the start line with anyone who will be with you or who is helping get you there.

○ **4 days:** Shop for day-before and race-morning foods.

○ **3 days:** Reminder: eat well, hydrate, keep off your feet.

○ **2 days:** Get a good night's sleep. It's actually more important to get a good night's sleep two days before race day than it is the night before, which might come as a relief to those of you who toss and turn the night before a race. If this is you, don't try to force sleep. Watch TV, read a book, meditate, clean. You can sleep when you're through the race.

○ **1 day:** Pick up your bib! Check out the expo! Look through your race bag one more time. Charge your watch. Keep your feet up, watch TV, read, and try to relax.

Race Morning

Wake up

Drink coffee

Eat breakfast

Drink water

Poop (If you need help with this, please check out Meghan Kita's book *How to Make Yourself Poop.*)

Get dressed and pin number on

Eat a light snack

Brush teeth

Depart for start line

Bag drop

Scope out porta-potties

Arrive at start line

Dynamic warm-up

Sip water

Use porta-potty
Fire up watch
Find your corral
Wish other racers good luck
Visualize race
Start!!!

WHAT IF YOU'RE NOT READY?

Unless there is an extreme extenuating circumstance like the story I'm about to tell you, then you are ready. If you've followed the training plans in here and put in the work, then you are ready. If you are nervous, remember you have nothing to be afraid of and remind yourself that you are ready. But if you are reading this because you have a suspicion that something is physically wrong, I understand. I've been there, and it ended in marathon heartache.

It was during that first marathon training cycle that I told you about early on in this book—the one I wish I could forget, the one where I jumped into in-season training way too quickly. Even though I was very young (late twenties) and fit, there was no way my bones could handle the load of the training plan I chose. But I didn't know that at the time and I consulted *zero* coaches and *zero* experts.

I had secret goals. I was new to working at *Runner's World*, surrounded by very fast veteran marathoners, and I thought I needed to prove myself. It was month two of my time as an editor there, and I became obsessed with the fact that I was one of the few runners on staff who had not run a marathon. What would happen if I didn't run one soon? Perhaps I would be fired! "If I don't run a marathon," I thought, "I am a fraud." I ignored the fact that my strength was always middle distance on the track—a far cry from 26.2 miles. Nope, not only did I need to run a marathon, I needed to run what I thought was a "respectable" time. As I stared into the abyss of pace charts, I decided that if I didn't break four hours, I would be laughed out of the office. (Let me stop here to tell my slower runners who may be reading: Anywhere near four hours is no joke. Simply finishing is more than respectable. Finishing in less than five hours is incredible for recreational athletes. Finishing under four hours? *Brava!*)

Nobody made me feel this way, but I was overwhelmed by the running-working culture. I mean, we literally did our weekly speed workouts on Wednesdays at lunch. I worked alongside Boston qualifiers and Olympic Trials qualifiers. I knew that realistically I wouldn't BQ in that first race, and I could deal with that. But I thought if I could just cross the finish in under four hours, I would be well on my way there! Or at least it would give my colleagues the illusion that I had real running potential.

As I write this, I realize how absurd my thought process was at the time. I let an extrinsic goal dictate everything I did during that training cycle. I ignored the advice from my amazing colleague Coach Meghan (the infamous hot dog marathoner). When I told her I was going to run a marathon, she not only invited me to join her on her long runs but offered tons of tips that I desperately needed. This was the first time she told me not to be a slave to the training plan. When she said it to me, I didn't really hear her. Instead, I nodded blankly, not understanding. Not only was I a slave to that dreaded twelve-week PDF, I added a few two-a-days, ran my repeats and intervals too fast, and of course, I wasn't strength training.

I made it to the taper with aches and pains. I thought that was normal, and for the most part the little discomfort I felt was pretty standard. More than anything, though, I was so relieved to make it to the final weeks. Training had become grueling, and the thought of having fewer miles to run felt overwhelmingly awesome.

A week away from the race, while out on a three-miler, I felt a crunch in my right shoe. I tried to ignore it, but shortly after the initial crunch, there was a sudden pain. I went through the first three stages of grief all at once, and inside my head, it sounded like this: "No, that's nothing—motherf*cker—if I can just get to the race I promise I will be a better person—no it's really nothing, forget it." I really did try to forget it. I denied that anything was wrong and I told no one.

Over the course of the next week, the pain only got worse. Finally, a day before I was set to travel to DC for the race, I hobbled into my supervisor's office. Katie, a superhuman runner mom with a generous heart, would know what to do. She was all-knowing when it came to fitness and injury recovery. I could hardly hold back tears when I started to tell her that I thought my foot was broken. "I'm so embarrassed," I said. Why would injury ever equate to weakness? I don't know. But like I said, I was young and kind of oblivious to how common these issues can be in the lead-up to a marathon. I asked her if she thought there was a way to tape my foot so it wouldn't hurt. She laughed. She called in a favor and got me squeezed in to see her podiatrist that night.

"You know," Katie said as I thanked her, "there are other races."

But I couldn't *not* run. I had to race and I had to run as fast as I could. I told Katie that dropping out was out of the question. When she asked me why, I couldn't articulate a response. But not running felt like my world would end. I'd poured every ounce of energy into this race. And what would people think?

I drove to the doctor's office that night after work. It was about forty-five minutes away, on the darkest roads in Pennsylvania, up and down foothills, winding through cow pastures and Amish country. When I finally made it to the office, I was shaking. I ripped my shoe off and showed the doctor my throbbing, swollen foot. There was no bruising, but it was a blob of hurt.

"When is the race?" he asked.

"Four days."

"When do you leave?"

"Tomorrow."

He is a runner, so thankfully he understood how much I thought was at stake. There was no time to get an MRI. He thought it could be plantar fasciitis or an entrapped nerve or a small stress fracture in one of the teeny tiny bird bones that make up our feet. But a diagnosis wasn't going to help—unless, of course, I wanted to wait for another race. "Philly is in three weeks," he offered. "You won't lose much. You can do some pool running."

I shook my head. Blasphemy. He understood. He taped my foot and showed me how to retape it. Ice and Advil, he said. Stay off it. He even gave me a steroid to keep with me if it got unbearable during the race. He understood because runners are insane. But, my dear marathoning friend, if something like this is happening to you, I need you to hear what I learned. There is always another race. If you compete unprepared, injured, or with any sort of doubt in your brain, you will not perform at your best.

By the grace of God, I finished that race. I was nearly hysterical at the end—and not just because I ran a 4:01, two minutes over my secret goal time, though that hurt too. My foot was wrecked. I'd basically skip-hopped the final three miles because the stabbing pain took over my entire body.

Looking back, I realize that my coworkers wouldn't have cared if I postponed my marathon. In fact, I don't think they would've minded if I stuck to 5Ks. They certainly did not care what time I ran. I placed an undue amount of pressure on myself and my poor little foot, and I nearly ruined the sport of the marathon for myself.

Way too many of us think that "no pain, no gain" is the driving philosophy of a fulfilling running life. But this is just not true. Being honest and kind to yourself is what will keep you in this running game.

My foot healed in time, though it still occasionally cramps up, as if to remind me of the pain I put it through all those years ago. My ego and the devastation I suffered from not achieving my time goal recovered only recently, when I discovered my actual running motivation.

It took five years, but when I sat down and thought about why people run marathons—why *I* run marathons—and I could articulate a reason that was not a time goal or an extrinsic goal of any kind—that was when I could put that dumb 4:01 behind me. I run not to prove my toughness to myself or others but to enjoy the feeling of strength and freedom it gives to me. So if during my next training cycle, my foot breaks ten days before the race, you better believe I'll wait for another marathon to come around. I encourage you to do the same. Being gritty is not being stupid. Being gritty is being determined to do your best in the face of challenges. Sometimes performing at your peak means listening to your body and having a little patience.

CHAPTER 12

IT'S STRATEGY TIME!

used to believe that you didn't need a race strategy. My plan was simply to finish, by any means necessary. But that's not the most effective method if you want to run your best race. And remember, even if this is your first marathon, if you put in the training, you want to run at your peak. Being smart and thinking about how to run the race in the weeks before the marathon will make you feel more prepared, which will allow your body to relax. As you think about how you will run the race, imagine it like you're downloading the information so that your legs and lungs can access it when they need to.

There are several ways to look at race strategy. Pace, racecourse features, small goals throughout the course—there are many things to consider. So let's figure this out!

THE GREAT SPLIT DEBATE

Pacing is the most obvious way to plan out the race. I often see runners lining up with a sort of temporary tattoo on one of their arms. It's a two-column chart with each mile listed and a corresponding time next to that mile. When I first saw these, I thought it was brilliant! Like, wow, if you just write down the time you're gonna run each mile in, you can just do it and hit your time goal.

Then I remembered how races work. Even if you know every hill, every water stop, every turn, and every pothole on the course, you cannot predict how you will run each mile on race day. Think about it: At the beginning of a marathon, we get trapped in corrals like sheep until our time group is ready to take off. If it's a really big race, we get stuck bobbing up and down for the first mile just trying to find a path, with little control of our pace and a lot of trapped energy. (This is good to know, newbies. You will hardly believe it when you hit the first mile! It's just a mob moving as one for that first stretch.) Once we hit mile two and the road starts to open up, even if we are cognizant of our energy expenditure, we run a little more swiftly than we wanted. Which, if I have mile times tattooed on me, might make me start doing running math (e.g., "If I ran a 10:10 when I was supposed to run a 9:20 and then 8:20 when I was supposed to run 9:45, I'm supposed to run mile three in . . . Wait, am I in mile three right now?"). That's a slippery slope, friends. The opposite of the zone. And literally anything could happen to knock you seconds off the assigned time. A puppy could start running alongside you! Your shoe could fall off. You might need a bathroom break. There might be a backwind so strong that you crush several miles effortlessly. So that's why I'm not a fan of getting that granular when it comes to pacing.

Runners often talk about splits, which are defined as a race's total time divided into smaller parts. For example, an even split means running at the same pace through an entire race. A positive split means running the first half of a race faster than the second half. A negative split means running the second half of the race faster than the first half. Most of the time when runners are discussing splits, they look at the race in two halves. Exercise scientists have studied pacing in the marathon ad nauseam. The most recent research asserts that even splits are most effective for amateur runners. As with anything, though, you have to choose what you feel most comfortable doing. There are pluses and minuses to the various methods, so let's talk it through.

Negative Splits

Many runners live by the negative-split philosophy, which means you run the first half of the race slower than the second half. It makes logical sense. You conserve energy in the first part of the race. Then, in the second half, you should have fuel left in the tank. For elite women, it seems to be the key to running strong.

Researchers at the Institute of Sport and Exercise Science at the University of Worcester looked at results from the women's marathon event at the 2009 IAAF World Athletics Championships and found that the top 25 percent of the field ran the first 10K at slower than their average pace. Twenty-two miles in, they increased their speed to above the average.

So the casual takeaway is that if the runner can hold back just enough for the early miles, she can really let loose on the last few. This method works really well for some, especially very experienced runners. If you know what your paces feel like and what your maximum effort is at various times of the race, then you will likely know how to push up against that barrier without saving too much in the beginning or burning out at any point.

For less experienced runners, it's hard to know if you're saving too much. Or you could concentrate so much on the time and pace in the first 10K that you burn the energy you meant to save. Plus, it takes tremendous discipline to go out slower than what you've considered "race pace" in the early miles of a marathon. You will have adrenaline bursting out of you—you will get swept up by the crowds! Remember, elites have the open road to work with, and often form a lead pack. They use each other to pace off, which is why we shouldn't necessarily make decisions based on their performance.

The edge we gain, if we successfully hold back in the beginning, might not amount to faster miles at the end. You will have still run more than twenty miles by the time you're supposed to speed up. The miles only get harder the farther you go. It's hard to know if you'll be able to really push on your way to the finish.

Positive Splits

When Mary Keitany ran the women-only marathon world record time of 2:17:01 in London in 2017, it was a positive split of more than three minutes. She ran 1:06:54 for her first half and 1:10:07 for her second. She broke away from the lead pack and ran a blistering third mile in 4:37. Nobody, including her training partners and the competitors closest to her, thought she could maintain the paces she was running. Her game plan was to beat Paula Radcliffe's women-only marathon time of 2:17:42, and Keitany used Radcliffe's paces as a sort of guide. Some analysts thought that she might've been aiming for Radcliffe's outright world record time (2:15:25 in a race that included men), which would've explained the incredible speed at which she took the first half and a sort of falling off that pace in the second. It was a risky maneuver but one that got her results.

So that's one time where positive splitting had a happy ending. For the rest of us, this can be referred to as the crash-and-burn method. The runners who use this method think that they should surge ahead and use their energy and fresh legs while they can. And ya know, for 5Ks, that can be really effective. But a marathon is 26.2 freaking miles, and if you go out at a pace that is too fast, you are bound to hurt in the latter part of the race. Most coaches will advise against attempting a positive split. I mean, if you're a live-hard-die-young kind of person and you can stomach the thought of pain for the last ten miles, go for it.

Even Splits

Studies show that women—at least nonelite women—are better suited for even pacing. One study looked at data from fourteen U.S. marathons that happened in 2011. Regardless of age and running experience, it found that women were more likely than men to maintain their running pace throughout a marathon and less likely to slow down in the second half of the race. This is good news!

If you want to compare yourself to an elite, then Des Linden should be your guiding light. Linden was called "the human metronome" by one Twitter fan because she consistently runs even splits in her marathons. In Boston 2017, she ran a perfect 1:12:33 for the first half and a 1:12:33 for the second. She is rarely off by more than a few seconds.

When following this method, your pace per mile should feel easy at the beginning and even into the second half of the marathon. You want the effort to feel easy for as long as possible. By the end, it should feel challenging but not impossible. Lack of experience will crush you if you go too fast too soon. Keep it steady, and the end result will likely exceed your expectations.

PACE GROUPS

Most races will give you the option of joining a pace group. So if you have a set time you think you will finish (e.g., 5:00), you can find pacers, who are usually wearing specific T-shirts and carrying a sign up high with the pace-group time listed on it.

If you are going for a PR and you enjoy other runners around you going for the same goal, then give this a shot. It gives you the opportunity to not worry about the times, paces, and miles. You can just relax and let go. Your pacers will likely take you on an even-split journey. They are experienced runners who know how to get to the finish running very consistently.

However, check in with them about their game plan well before the gun goes off. If they tell you that they plan to negative split, but you want to go out quicker than the time they propose, then ditch 'em. You can also use a pace group for a segment of the race and break off to fall back or pull ahead at any time. Don't feel like you're married to them.

It's an incredible feeling to cross with a group of people all aiming for the same time. Plus, pacers can be incredible sources of inspiration and can pull you through the dark times. I've run races both with pace groups and solo. It depends on my goals for the race and my mood on the day.

DETAILS

Finally, make some decisions that might seem like afterthoughts well in advance. Ask yourself the following, and plan accordingly:

1. If it is cold or rainy, will I wear a sweatshirt or poncho (advised) to the start? At what point will I throw this away? Newbies, many runners wear an outer layer, gloves, maybe a hat to the start of a race to stay warm and dry and keep muscles loose. They toss off these garments, usually before the end of the first mile. Don't expect to see these clothes again—they are usually donated or thrown away.

2. Am I going to walk through water stations? Some runners refuse to walk at all during the race. Other runners want to take time to make sure they get the hydration and nutrition they need without it spilling down the front of them. Do what you've been doing during your long runs.

3. Do I know the course well? Do I know where the turns are? If you are aiming for a PR, study the course so you know where you will be turning. Crossing the road to prepare for the curve can shave seconds off your time.

While having a pace for each mile might be misguided for some, knowing how you will approach each mile or different segments of the course is helpful for your mental game. It's especially important if you can't seem to focus, feel a little off at the start, or experience an unprecedented amount of anxiety.

You want to run the mile you're in. That will give you the best chance of finding your groove. If merely reminding yourself of that Zen mode isn't enough, make small goals for each mile. They do not have to be overly complicated. In fact, the simpler the better. And even if you make twenty-six goals, you do not need to think of them all or use them in the order you put them down. They are meant to pull your attention to the moment, make you feel at ease, and provide the satisfaction of a mini accomplishment. For example, in the first mile, my goal is to keep my breath steady. The excitement and anticipation might try to creep in and make my breath uneven, so I lock in a nice, even breath. In the second mile, I want to find a part of the road I like and try to stay in that lane. In the third mile, I will focus on my cadence and make an effort to feel light on my feet.

Race Strategy Worksheet

What is my *why*?

_____

_____

_____

_____

What are my overall goals?

_____

_____

_____

_____

Average race pace:

_____

_____

Power word:

_____

_____

I am most excited about:

_____

_____

_____

_____

I plan to run_____splits

What can I accomplish each mile?

Mile 1		Mile 14	
Mile 2		Mile 15	
Mile 3		Mile 16	
Mile 4		Mile 17	
Mile 5		Mile 18	
Mile 6		Mile 19	
Mile 7		Mile 20	
Mile 8		Mile 21	
Mile 9		Mile 22	
Mile 10		Mile 23	
Mile 11		Mile 24	
Mile 12		Mile 25	
Mile 13		Mile 26	

CHAPTER 13

YOU CAN DO IT

Dear friend, read this the night before the race. Ultimately, the marathon is you versus yourself. You, facing down 26.2 miles and getting through them no matter what. I can't get you to the finish line, but you don't need me. The only thing you need is the knowledge of how capable you are. Once you get to the other side, you will look back at your race and realize how far you've come and how much work it took to get there. You will have done it on your own. You will have conquered goals and become stronger than you have ever been before. Imagine that scene. Imagine yourself looking back at the months of training, and imagine feeling that pride. Let that pride wash over you like a glowing light, and smile and breathe and know that this feeling is just hours away.

Think about where you started in this process. Close your eyes for a moment and remember the first mile you ran with the intention of finishing the marathon you're running tomorrow. You've come so far. You've trained to become the best version of yourself. You've shown extraordinary discipline and made enormous sacrifices. Because of your determination, you are going to shine. Trust your training. You've got this. If the race gets hard, embrace it. Remind yourself:

It's supposed to be hard.
You love the challenge.
You love running.

Now visualize yourself at the start, surrounded by other runners. Fix your eyes straight ahead, beyond the first timing mat, out onto the course, and take a deep breath in. Thank your body for its sacrifices and its strength. Bring your shoulders back, exhale. Think about what you want to accomplish. Your legs are fresh and ready to go. Your lungs feel clear, your breath is calm. You are tough. When you unlock the strength inside you tomorrow, the road will open before you and you will know that everything is possible. Everything you need is in your heart.

CHAPTER 14

BEYOND THE RACE

You've crossed the finish line. You grabbed your race medal, hobbled away from the corral with your space blanket draped over your shoulders, stood triumphantly in a sea of other finishers, and likely thought to yourself, "When do I get to sit down?"

Now that you have mastered the marathon, what is next? What do you do in the minutes, hours, days, and weeks following your big finish? I will break it down for you step by step, because this is an important time for your mind and your body.

MINUTES AFTER FINISHING

You might make it to the end and feel like you're on cloud nine. You might make it and collapse into a ball on the pavement and have to be scooped up like roadkill by race officials. No matter what category you fall into, there are three important things to do immediately after you cross the line.

First, get warm. You might feel too hot to cover yourself with the metallic blanket, but my friend, this silver covering is a lifesaver. As soon as you stop moving, your body temperature will decrease quite rapidly because your muscles have stopped working. The technology in these things is incredible. This blanket will keep heat in, regulate your body temperature, and prevent you from catching a chill. This is important, since it might be several minutes before you get to dry clothes. When you do get to your gear bag or your marathon spectator buddy who is holding a fresh change of clothing, try to strip off your sweaty stuff ASAP. You might not be in the right head space to make this decision, so tell someone to remind you to take care of yourself.

Second, begin rehydrating. Hopefully you stuck to your race hydration routine, but you're likely still very depleted. Now is the time to get fluids in. Snag a water bottle and a sports drink if your race provides them at the end. If you can stomach it, try to eat a little something. Bananas are a delicious and nutritious option. Pretzels or other salty snacks can help regulate your fluids. You might not be hungry yet, but you will be ravenous later. No matter their best efforts, some people experience dehydration or hyponatremia. If you're feeling unwell, dizzy, or faint, or you're cramping like crazy (like your legs are stiff and you cannot walk), go to the medical tent. It's always better to be safe. They can give you IV fluids and you'll be on your way to recovery.

Third, soak in this moment. You just did something that most people only dream about completing. Thank your legs. Thank your body. Call someone special. Hug the people at the race with you. Don't be afraid to cry. You might want to sob tears of joy or you might be in postrace agony! Feel it all! Take a few mental snapshots. It will be hard to duplicate this feeling—every finish is different, and every finish is remarkable in its own way. Now might be a good time to think about your *why*, the thing that kept you going all these weeks. Embrace the feeling of success and accomplishment. You have achieved so much.

HOURS AFTER FINISHING

OK, not to be too alarmist, but try not to be alone for at least eight hours after finishing. Your body put in a lot of work and it might start rebelling. You might pass out, or get dizzy, or just be a little foggy. Driving isn't the best idea. You might feel extraordinarily tired and just not yourself at all. That's normal. Here are some must-dos to lessen the marathon hangover.

Keep moving, but just a little bit. A slow walk will work wonders for you.

Walk for ten to fifteen minutes within the hour after finishing the race. Do a slow walk every three or so hours for the rest of the day.

Stretch lightly. Let your body tell you what can and cannot be stretched. Gently move your limbs, but resist the urge to turn yourself inside out. A nice supine twist, some neck rolls, a few calf flexes—that's what should be on the agenda for the day. If you plan to foam-roll, wait at least six hours after the race.

Elevate your legs. Put those poor feet up for fifteen minutes to reduce inflammation.

Eat. You know, if you eat the right recovery foods after the race, then you will feel like a rock star in the days ahead. But if you want a doughnut, eat a doughnut. Just make sure you add good proteins, fats, and carbs to your plate as well.

Shower using cool or lukewarm water. Wait a few days before soaking in a hot tub. The heat might cause inflammation and slow down muscle recovery.

Nap, sleep, relax. Do your best to chill out and get some good rest. This will give your body the best chance to heal.

THE WEEK FOLLOWING THE RACE

In the days immediately following the race, you will probably have some muscle soreness. Going down stairs and attempting to sit on a toilet seat will require extra time and probably cause a lot of grunting and even some swearing. Treat these aches with pain relievers, slow walking, rest, foam-rolling, and a very gentle massage.

Many runners will fall into a funk. Your mood might plummet. Exhaustion and sadness are totally normal for the week after a race. Your life might feel empty without the anticipation of the race. You will have much more time on your hands and the initial glee of finishing will be gone. Ugh. I wish I could say this won't happen to you, but the truth is, it's hard to predict or prevent. Instead, plan for it. Treat yourself. Maybe your running shoes are toasted—get yourself a new pair. Do something nice for yourself that is non–running related. Do you like manicures? Go to the salon. Eat healthy meals, including brain- and mood-boosting foods like salmon, walnuts, fruits, and veggies. About three days after, you can bathe, so relax and enjoy a wonderful spa experience right in your own home. But most important, be kind to yourself and your feelings. Remind yourself that you are allowed to feel sad. This feeling will pass.

Many runners will start training again three or so days after the race. It's fine to do so, as long as you ease into it and as long as you feel ready to run. If you go out and try and find that your legs are still heavy and sore, just walk. Healing is your priority right now.

That being said, if you're ready to go, the best plan is to do the reverse taper. So go back to your marathon plan and look at the last three weeks. Do them in reverse. This will gradually build you back up and set you up well for maintenance mode.

Maintenance is that time between races when you are just keeping up your fitness. After a marathon, you are in extraordinary shape. Many coaches will tell you not to waste that and to maintain it by running an average number of miles until you want to base train again. This will keep you ready for base level, so you don't have to go all the way through pre-base again. Depending on how you feel, you could even jump into the second month of base training and focus on plyometric strength to gain some additional speed.

The thing is, you don't *have* to jump right into maintenance mode if you don't want to. You won't lose your current fitness level for two weeks. Also, it's totally fine to be sick of running. Even if you're not sick of running, you might want to consider taking a short break to completely recover mentally and physically.

So what does that look like? It's a two-week recovery period. This is an opportunity to cut your weekly miles (as dictated by the taper) in half. Or you could choose to not run at all. That doesn't mean you should sit on your couch and watch Netflix, though I wouldn't fault you if you did. Instead, go on leisurely walks. Try swimming or gentle yoga. Recovering fully will only get you stronger for your next race. When you're done with your two-week recovery period, do the reverse taper. You will probably feel just as strong as you did in the week leading up to the race.

WHEN SHOULD I RACE AGAIN?

This is the golden question, friend. I know marathoners who get to the finish line and start thinking about the next 26.2 they want to run. I've known a friend to sign up for their next race on the shuttle ride back from the finish line. I know another friend who missed her PR by seconds and decided to sign up to run another race two weeks later so she could reap the benefits of her current fitness level. (I advise against this, by the way.) There are other runners who take years between marathons. And yet others who never run the full distance ever again.

There is no right answer. It will be whatever is right for you. But when you're thinking about running your next race, remember the first steps you took at the start of this journey. Why do you want to race again? Will that reason get you to the finish stronger than before? Can you dedicate yourself to the process? What does base training look like this time around? Are you committed to getting stronger, faster, and smarter?

If you have the answers to these questions, and I'm sure you do, then get ready. It's time to master the marathon all over again.

ACKNOWLEDGMENTS

Thank you to the incredible Amy Sun for helping to make this book as great as it could be. Thank you, Linda Konner, for believing in the idea of a guide for women and helping me at every turn. And thank you, James Jayo, for recognizing the importance of a book like this and refining the initial concept. Thanks to Des Linden for your incredible words and inspiration to all female athletes. To all elite women marathoners—you elevate the women's running community every day.

Thank you to my incredible husband, Bryan Croot, who is my everything. He helped me plan, proofread, brainstorm, and run throughout the writing process. My animals, Ollie, Gus, and Kiki, deserve some credit. Though they cannot read, they listened as I read sentences aloud.

My family, who may be the most supportive people on the planet, have been with me every step of the way: my mom, Connie Nolan; Ursula, Keith, Ferris, and Willa Berg; Victoria Nolan; Maria Campo; Lucy Campo; Joe Annecharico; Carolyn and Rich Marcolus; Tony Campo; Ronnie Vazquez; Maria and Paul Kolarsick; Alan and Ann Nolan; Rod and Diane Lenniger; Penni and Bob Croot; Taryn and Rory Weinstein; Michele Croot; Loryn Croot; and all my cousins and extended family. I am grateful every day to have your support and love.

My very best running friends: Meghan Kita, Heather Mayer Irvine, Hannah McGoldrick, and Danielle Zickl, what would I even do without you? Thank you for your advice, wisdom, motivation, and general awesomeness. Also, thank you, Matt Damon, who makes all things possible. To my experts—Kaci Brandt, Heather Caplan, Erica Coviello, Hillary Israelsen, Mary Johnson, Ashlee Lawson Green, Ellen London, Dez McQueen, Dan Moody, Kirstin Ritchie, and Crystal Seaver—no one would be able to master a marathon without you.

Thank you, *Runner's World* family, especially Matt Allyn, John Atwood, Erin Benner, Derek Call, Budd Coates, Brian Dalek, Dave Graf, John Hanc, Kit Fox, Riley Missel, Katie Neitz, Kristen Parker, Suzanne Perreault, Taylor Rojek, Bill Strickland, David Willey, and Bart Yasso. Thank you to my incredible teammates at Utah Valley University: Christie Denniston and Lindsay Watson.

Thank you to my grandpa, Anthony Campo; my uncle, Phil Campo; and my father, Chuck Nolan, who are my guardian angels. I know they helped me finish this book! And thank you, God.